THE OTHER
MEDICINES

Books by Richard Grossman

BOLD VOICES

CHOOSING & CHANGING

THE OTHER MEDICINES

THE OTHER MEDICINES

Richard Grossman

DOUBLEDAY & COMPANY, INC.
GARDEN CITY, NEW YORK
1985

LIBRARY OF CONGRESS CATALOGING IN PUBLICATION DATA

Grossman, Richard L. (Richard Lee), 1921–
    The other medicines.
        Bibliography: p. 195
        Includes index.
    1. Therapeutics, Physiological.   I. Title.
    RM700.G76   1985   615.5   80-2857
            ISBN 0-385-15834-3
            ISBN 0-385-15835-1 (pbk.)

For my daughters,

Joan, Nancy, and Lucy

Men, in fact, desire from science nothing else but the benefits; not the arguments, but the definitions. Accordingly, our intention in this book is to shorten long-winded discourses and synthesize the various ideas. Our intention also, however, is not to neglect the advice of the ancients.

Ibn Botlan, "the Physician,"
from the preface to the
Tacuinum Sanitatis
(15th century)

CONTENTS

ACKNOWLEDGMENTS

For the past ten years I have been a member of the faculty of the Residency Program in Social Medicine and the Department of Family Medicine at Montefiore Medical Center, working both as part of the psychosocial faculty and as director of the Health in Medicine Project, a research and education effort devoted to studying the possible integration of complementary therapies into primary medical care for patients in ambulatory care settings.

My greatest debt, therefore, is to the residents—internists, pediatricians, and family physicians—who have trained in this program, and to my faculty colleagues. As my teachers, my students, my preceptors, my associates, and above all, as my friends, they have been ideal companions: critical and challenging as well as encouraging and supportive. At the sites in which these physicians practice—the Valentine Lane Family Practice, the Dr. Martin Luther King Jr. Health Center, the Family Health Center—I have had the priceless opportunity to work with them and their patients, and see at first hand both the difficulties and the opportunities inherent in any attempt to synthesize widely various medical approaches.

Many others have been of immense help to me, both directly and indirectly, in the writing of this book. I thank especially: Walter Anderson, José Aponte, D.Ac., Susan McMillan Arensberg, William B. Bateman, M.D., Rabbi Leonard Beerman, Bill Binzen, Harrison G. Bloom, M.D., Patricia S. Bloom, M.D., Jo Ivey Boufford, M.D., Mariada and Simon Bourgin, Stephen Chang, M.D., Chung-liang Al Huang, Fredeswilda Cintron, Harris Coulter and Catherine Coulter, David B. Eagle, M.D., Marji Gold, M.D., Robert B. Greifinger, M.D., Leon Hammer, M.D., Professor Wayland Hand, Luis Hernandez, Mildred Jackson, Jacques Jovanny, M.D., Daniel E. Korin, M.D., Cynthia Lanahan, Didier Maillot, Robert J. Massad, M.D., Claudio Naranjo, M.D., Ni Hua Ching, M.D., Dr. Nathan Novick, Naomi Rabinowitz, M.D., Robert Schiller, M.D., Mitchell Schorrow, John Shen, M.D., Frances Siegel, M.D., Pat Shonubi, R.N., Michael Smith, M.D., David Sobel, M.D., A. H. Strelnick, M.D., Dana Ullmann, Laura S. Welch, M.D., Andrew Weil, M.D., Harold Wise, M.D., and the Vicki List Zelman Fund.

In connection with the actual publication of this book, I have had the help of a gifted group of publishing people: Robert Lescher, Randall Greene, William Strachan, and Nancy Tuckerman all gave me support along the way, while Samuel Vaughan and James Moser provided the wise editorial guidance and assistance that ultimately made the book possible. Thanks, too, to my friends Maria Falcon and Judy Fawcett for their work on the preparation of the manuscript.

Much of the work on Part II, "Natural First Aid," is also part of a manual prepared for the use of the practitioners in the Dr. Martin Luther King Jr. Health Center, the Valentine Lane Family Practice, and the Family Health Center. An enthusiastic and skillful team was involved in that work and are thus responsible for much of the organization and content of this book as well. My enduring thanks go to them all: Sybil Lefferts, Janice Caldwell, Marie Conte, Catherine O'Halloran, and, again, the faculty and resident physicians of the Residency Program in Social Medicine and the Department of Family Medicine.

Finally, as in all my work—and my life—my primary collaborator is my wife, Ann Arensberg, to whom I owe thanks that cannot be expressed in words.

East Arlington, Vermont
August 1984

AUTHOR'S NOTE

A waggish friend of mine once suggested that this book carry the subtitle *Thirteen New Ways to Stop a Nosebleed.* That phrase does capture at least part of the spirit of the book's contents, which include a number of substances, exercises, body manipulations, "pressure points," postures, and improvised devices drawn from unorthodox medical systems to help alleviate a number of common distressing symptoms ranging from abrasions to toothaches. But I have a further intention beyond wanting to describe the self-treatments that form Part II of this book, "Natural First Aid."

In the narrative chapters that precede that manual, I attempt to explain the history, theory, and practice of a number of medical systems that, although they lie outside the establishment we think of as scientific medicine, nevertheless have much to offer those who are ill or injured. I believe that the more we understand the principles and techniques of these medical traditions, the more we will find them compatible with "our" system—the Western scientific medicine that has developed over the past one hundred years in association with laboratory research. That consensual medicine is truly a remarkable scientific enterprise, but it is not the only body of thought and experience that may contribute to the relief of human pain or discomfort, and while I think there is no reason to repeal or abandon the gains of scientific medicine, I also feel there is every reason to expand and enlarge it to include other forms of treatment and healing. I believe we are entitled to the most comprehensive vision of health and medicine of which the human mind is capable, and in my work in medical education and clinical practice, I have seen the marvelous ways in which systems as disparate as acupuncture and chemotherapy, herbal medicines and complex surgery, Yogic meditation and physiotherapy, breathing exercises and psychiatry can work together in a complementary way to provide greater benefits to ailing persons than any one of those treatments might provide alone.

This book, then, is not about medical systems that are alternatives to "our" medicine, but about those that I believe make the greatest demands for inclusion in both orthodox medical practice and self-treatment. For the most part, I have described the way these other medicines are used for symptomatic complaints, so that the "Natural First Aid" section of the book does not deal with "alternative" or unconventional treatments for conditions such as arthritis, cancer, cardiovascular disease, and so on, although during the course of such serious diseases or chronic illnesses, a number of secondary symptoms may occur which are eminently treatable with the procedures I have described here.

Obviously, I have not described the theory and practice of all the "other" medicines. I have not included, for example, a number of systems that I believe to merit serious consideration, but that I consider either too specialized for ready inclusion in conventional medical practice or not easily suited to self-care without extensive training. Consider: hypnosis, particularly of the kind taught and practiced by Milton H. Erickson, which has established itself firmly as one of the most useful therapies available in many situations: impulse control (for the obese, or the cigarette smoker), chronic headaches, intractable pain, and for the management of stress and tension; the Alexander technique, a remarkably useful "reeducation of the body," that has helped thousands of victims of musculoskeletal problems; the movement and body awareness methods of Moshe Feldenkrais that give a new meaning to the principle of mind-body correlations; the Bates method of developmental vision therapy that has enabled many people to forego their need for eyeglasses and help others to maintain their normal vision; the Bach flower remedies, a group of thirty-eight preparations made from flowering trees and plants that have been used successfully in England and the United States, in a manner similar to the action of homeopathic preparations, and are credited with treating both emotional and physical disorders; and aeriontherapy, which uses an air ionizer to produce an increase in negative ions in the immediate environment, with the consequence that many people suffering from respiratory ailments, rheumatism, migraine headaches, heart palpitations, and allergic reactions such as hayfever are substantially relieved of their symptoms. The Annotated Bibliography at the end of this book includes references to a number of books about these systems, and may be helpful in leading interested readers to further information about them.

In addition, I have not included full descriptions of a number of systems and methods that I have come to believe are of little or no relevance to the subject of this book, even though some of them may contain principles or details that could help relieve suffering: radionics, radiesthesia, reflexology (zone therapy), cranial massage, iridology, psionic medicine, hydrotherapy, aroma therapy, color therapy, Do-in, megavitamin therapy, pyramid therapy, and sound therapy.

As to the systems you *will* read about in this book, I am a convert to none of them and a believer in all of them. I believe that each of these medical doctrines has something helpful to offer those who suffer; I believe that none is based on mere superstition or occult principles; I believe that each has survived not simply because of temporal or cultural faith in them; I believe that each is a bona fide part of human knowledge and, as such, belongs to all of us for our possible benefit.

Finally, although the recommendations in this book are confined to symptomatic relief, they are not meant to replace the first aid techniques of the *Standard First Aid and Personal Safety* manual prepared by the American Red Cross or the British St. John's Ambulance Brigade manual, but rather to provide an adjunctive, complementary source of things to do that might help mitigate pain, discomfort, or a threat to life. Whatever steps you take, it should be remembered that "first aid" describes the emergency treatment given to a stricken person before medical or surgical care can be administered by a trained individual. This definition emphasizes the point that all emergency measures should be accompanied or followed by professional treatment by a physician or other qualified health care practitioner.

PART I

THE OTHER MEDICINES

The role of medicine is to help man
function well as long as feasible, and
if possible, happily in all his endeavors—
whether he is toiling for his daily bread,
creating urban civilization, writing a poem,
or attempting to reach the moon. These
examples are not taken at random; they
symbolize that medicine relates to all
human activities, to the responses of man
in the worlds of nature, thought, feeling,
and technology.

René Dubos
Man, Medicine, and Environment

1.
ECUMENICAL MEDICINE

The most electrifying event of the fall of 1932 in Miss Ziegler's seventh-grade class in the Harrison Hill School in Fort Wayne, Indiana, was not the election of Franklin D. Roosevelt as President of the United States. That news, of course, was a subject of much discussion in civics class, but our imaginations were not half so fired by it as they were by what Lane McCord said to Miss Ziegler one morning in hygiene class. "My grandfather says a drop of piss is good for pinkeye." There it was, just as plain as you please, and it was as if Lane's voice had shot into the air like a Roman candle at Emerson Park on the Fourth of July. We all waited, slack-jawed, for the dazzling explosion to follow.

But Miss Ziegler simply ruffled a few papers, stood up erectly next to her desk, and spoke very quietly. "We call that *urine,*" she said, in a slow and even voice, "and yes, Lane, there are people who believe urine is helpful for eye irritations like pinkeye, which is really called conjunctivitis. Today doctors use boric acid drops for that." At the sound of the word "urine" there had been a few giggles and some shuffling of feet, but for the most part we remained gravely silent, our ears still ringing with Lane's prescription, and as Miss Ziegler went on to talk about eyecups and the blue bottles of collyrium that she told us were also good for the eyes, no one in the room could shake off the sound that dirty word had made.

Such were the standards of the time that our parents, too, would have been shocked at the public use of barnyard language in a classroom, but if they had ever heard of the use of urine as an eyewash, they would have been equally surprised that such lore persisted in twentieth-century Indiana, even within farm families like the McCords. Fort Wayne was a modern town, after all, though Dr. Salen still made housecalls when you had the measles or whooping cough. There was a well-known tuberculosis sanitarium on the north side, filled with doctors and nurses and equipment, and I had seen the mysterious instruments and test tubes of St. Joseph's Hospital when I had spent the night there following my tonsillectomy. (I had described in a paper for Miss Ziegler the dreamlike experience of inhaling ether through a black rubber mask.) No, in 1932 our parents were sure our town was not going to remain just the seat of a rural county; we were going to be in the vanguard of scientific progress. They were assembling more-and-more-sophisticated machinery at the General Electric plant, electrifying the gasoline pumps at the Wayne Pump factory, and my father had told me that someday on the Pennsylvania Railroad, for which he worked, there would be trains traveling at speeds of more than 150 miles an hour!

Both my parents were frail, and obsessed with the fear of serious illness. My father had spent six months in that "TB" sanitarium and had been warned that his lungs were not "strong," and my mother was convinced that her continuing racking cough at the evening dinner table was cancer, the word that was always whispered or said softly with a hand half covering the mouth. In my family, doctors of all kinds were revered and their suggestions taken as military commands; as a result, I went through an entire year ingesting a tablespoon of liquid iron every night to "build my blood," and on one occasion, when Dr. Salen suggested my occasional headaches might be the result of too much extracurricular reading, I was put on a strict quota of two books a week, and was reduced to smuggling out my other reading to a tar-paper-covered shack some older boys had built in the woods for the safekeeping of copies of the *Police Gazette* and their secret experiments with smoking (corn-silk cigarettes) and chewing (Red Man tobacco). Doctors were the arbiters of health, and health was neatly limited to the immediate and current state of your body, and in the case of children, the measurement of your height and weight against the norms of the day.

If my parents had known that both animal and human urine had a long history of use in medicine in Asia and Europe (twenty-five hundred years), both as an internal medication for certain respiratory conditions and fever, as well as a topical application for ulcers of the skin and to styes and other eye irritations, their reactions would have hovered between mockery and outrage. They were creatures of their times, committed to the idea that sheerly physical and material well-being was the north and south of progress, and that only the tangible and validated cures of hospital surgery, the latest drugs, and the injunctions of a certified physician (preferably a graduate of Harvard Medical School) could assure our health. So pervasive was that devotion that if one of my uncles reported casually that he had lost his job, my parents would respond, almost in unison, "Listen, George, things will be all right. As long as you have your health. . . ."

In the fifty years since Lane McCord's shocking suggestion in hygiene class, ideas about health and medicine have, along with almost every other trusted truism of the past, come in for broad and deep debate and considerable revision. Psychological and mental factors have been added to the physical model of health and illness, and, by extension, the environmental, cultural, and occupational influences on health have come to be recognized as centrally important. All the powers of physics and chemistry that thrust General Electric and Wayne Pump into advanced industrial success have been enlisted in the cause of medicine. Dr. Salen has been replaced by a battery of specialists who have divided human health into such refined and isolated segments that one criticism of modern medical practice is that doctors know "more and more about less and less."

The complaint against overspecialization has led, in turn, to other critiques. Modern medicine's religious reliance on technological forms of diagnosis and treatment; its air of depersonalization that leads to objectifying patients as mere vehicles for disease; its quick and often arrogant invasion of the human body with surgery or intervention with chemotherapy; its startling costs that have contributed so hugely to the broken back of the world economy, and excluded so many impoverished people from its technical miracles; its elitism and paternalism that has made the white, male, affluent doctor into a high priest dispensing to the children of the tribe—all these charges continue to be leveled at the practitioners of contemporary scientific medicine, even as many of my parents' visions are being realized through its remarkable achievements. That medicine, which anthropologists have come to call "cosmopolitan" medicine, in contrast to the indigenous "ethnomedicines" of Africa and Asia and the "folk medicines" of subcultures everywhere, has survived criticisms and remains politically and economically dominant today, though in absolute numbers it is a minority practice, because more people in the world are served by the treatments of "ethnic" or "popular" medicine.

Despite its statistical minority, however, scientific medicine remains so powerful that all other medical systems are known by their distinctions from it. They are thought of as antiestablishment, or, at best, nonestablishment. This has led to the spread of simplistic dichotomies such as "traditional versus modern," "primitive versus civilized," or "orthodox versus unorthodox," forms which have the subtle effect of making the unusual or uncommon medicines sound like senseless or amateur rebellions against accepted wisdom. Inevitably, any therapeutic approach that does not stem directly from the Western physics and chemistry that are the bedrock of cosmopolitan medicine is seen as occult, and is considered not only different, but inferior. Even more neutral terms used to describe these approaches have that same negative shading: "Fringe" medicine, "marginal" medicine, "alternative" medicine and, of course, "holistic" medicine, the most popular and least understood label for all that is outside standard, institutionalized Western medicine.

The use of the term "holistic" has become so loose and thoughtless that the term is virtually bankrupt and meaningless. Any moment now we'll see a chain of holistic doughnut shops. Possibly no legitimate, serious idea has gained such quick currency and, at the same time, such outrageous distortion.

The word "holism" was born in 1926, on page 99 of the book *Holism and Evolution,* written by Jan Christiaan Smuts, a man best known as a hero of the Boer War and as the first Prime Minister of the South Africa that emerged from that war. In Miss Ziegler's history class he was held up as a hero for his liberal, vigorous support of the League of Nations (though his less admirable role in the bargaining with Gandhi over the issue of racial discrimination in his country was never mentioned).

Smuts's book was the culmination of his lifetime study of biology. Since his college days at Cambridge he had been fascinated by the puzzle of biological evolution, and though his ultimate theory ranged far beyond biology into the realms of social organization, and included an elaborate and rather wrong-headed psychology of human personality he called "personology," the word he coined, "holism" (from the Greek *holos,* "whole"), was meant to convey his central idea. It was completely original and as radical as much of the "new physics" of his time. The heart of that concept was contained in two statements:

> The creation of wholes, and *even more highly organized wholes,* and of wholeness generally as characteristic of existence, is an inherent character of the universe . . . it marks the line of evolutionary progress. And Holism is the inner driving force behind that progress. . . .

> A *whole,* which is more than the sum of its parts, has something internal, some inwardness of structure and function, some specific inner relation, some internality of character or nature, which constitutes that *more.*

Though Smuts argued strenuously in the book that his theory explains cellular growth as surely as it explained the development of personality and social processes, his idea did not take root in biology. Rather, the holistic perspective, which saw the human organism in a "constant state of excitation," a dynamic striving toward "self-actualization," engaged the interest of psychologists dissatisfied by the neat and tidy explanations of Freud and the behaviorists. Such psychologists—primarily Kurt Goldstein (by training originally a biologist), and Abraham Maslow—seized on and expanded holistic theory and demonstrated that it offered a new definition of human nature. They attributed to that nature an inner, transcendent power not allowed for in theories that human beings, as the behaviorists would have it, were only reflexive, limited to responding in predictable and universal ways to external stimuli, or were, at best, as Freudian theory held, prisoners of their animal nature, capable of only "sublimating" their destructive tendencies and forming civilization by overcoming their repressions and their baser instincts.

Challenging these two dominant—and still dominant—philosophies of human nature also served to challenge the methods by which they were developed. Freudian and behaviorist ideas derived from analysis, the reduction and "atomizing" of parts of human behavior into manageable, small units and considering those parts in isolation from the organism as a whole. The analytical method is the foundation of science as it has developed, and the holistic theorists never denied this. Their argument was with the grandiose and comprehensive *conclusions* drawn from the information obtained by analysis, and with the dogged insistence of the static-analytic theorists that the behavior of parts explains the whole. The holistic camp wanted to explore the way the entire human being—his mind as well as his body, his powers of abstract thought as well as his ability to act in concrete ways, his capacities for innovation, spontaneity, and choice as well as his needs for food, safety, and shelter—could cope and grow in the environment of nature. From holism they derived a psychology of health and transcendence; they developed and legitimized the study of the innate strength of the human mind and body to complement the emphasis that conventional science had placed on the pathology and diseases with which that mind and body had to struggle. They included as part of the rightful agenda of psychology, biology, biochemistry, and medicine itself the issues of the human "spirit," values, potentialities for growth, love, and above all, the inherent power of the person to heal himself—the very process that even classical medicine has always acknowledged took place as part of medical "treatment."

The confluence of the holistic idea with the reemergence of Jungian psychology, the existential psychologies of Germany and France, the revival of interest in the Asian psychologies imbedded in the philosophies of Buddhism, Taoism, and Hinduism, the similar Renaissance of popularity of American Transcendentalism as espoused by Emerson, Thoreau, William James, and the inward-turning appetites of the restless American culture in the 1960s—all these came together to create the "human potential movement." Kurt Goldstein, Gordon Allport, Gardner Murphy, Carl Rogers, Rollo May, and Abraham Maslow were the psychologist-gods of it, and Martin Heidegger, Martin Buber, Aldous Huxley and Lewis Mumford gave it a literary and philosophical coloration. What most of us saw on the surface, of course, was the Esalen Institute—the paradisiacal blowout center on the cliffs of Big Sur, California, where nude marathon groups "encountered" in the moonlight, and the setting for psychotherapy appeared to have shifted from the couch to an outdoor circus under the eucalyptus trees. What is significant for our purposes, however, is that the theory behind the experimentation and exploration that went on in the Esalen "laboratory" (to put a generous construction on it), was *holistic* in principle. The "whole person"—not just the mind, with all its repressed traumas and its tendency to respond to stimulus, and not just the body, with its stored tensions and constrictions—was the target. Movement and manipulation systems which posited an exchange of con-

trol—mind over body, and the reverse—were integral parts of the training. Not surprisingly, little known or ancient systems like Hatha Yoga, the
Alexander technique, T'ai Chi Ch'uan, and Aikido became popular. New
systems in the same spirit were given equal emphasis: neo-Reichian
bioenergetics, Structural Integration (rolfing), polarity therapy and massage, clinical biofeedback training, Feldenkrais's "awareness through
movement," and others.

The human potential movement, which spread out from Esalen all
through the 1960s, became the host and umbrella for teachers and researchers in all these fields, and by 1970 holistic techniques involving the
body/mind graduated from an emphasis on relaxation or control of
movement to concern with what had previously been the purview of
medicine: the treatment—by other than conventional, Western scientific
means—of accidents, illness, and disease that threatened life itself. What
the holistic perspective provided was the idea of the possible fusion of
approaches: East and West, old and new, mental and physical, medical
and nonmedical.

At this point in the proliferation of the holistic idea there occurred a
branching into two streams of activity that, although they overlap and
crisscross in many ways, have differing emphases. On the one hand, those
whose main interest lay in what has been called the "promotive" aspects
of health linked up directly or indirectly with the "fitness craze" and
health consciousness that was already blossoming. Thus, macrobiotic nutrition teachers, citing the "holistic" spirit of their Buddhist background,
found the classical vegetarians and those involved in organic farming; the
health-making possibilities of dancing and painting, and even chanting,
were explored in more organized and disciplined ways; the meditative
quality of long-distance running and jogging suggested that mental as
well as muscle tone could be improved through exercise; training in such
previously taken-for-granted processes as breathing, sitting, standing,
and walking were discovered (or rediscovered) as means to emotional and
physical enhancement; the simple act of touching elaborated into a dozen
new schools of body massage, became a popular form of promoting
"whole health."

Simultaneous with this burgeoning movement, challenging the old
ideas of calisthenics, a "balanced diet," fresh air, and eight hours of sleep
with open windows as the only keys to health, another branch of the
holistic movement turned to the issue of curative medicine. It studied or
devised systems that, although they, too, addressed the whole person—
body, mind, spirit, and feelings—did so from the standpoint of healing
and curing distress as well as maintaining and promoting normal functions. Thus, in the early 1970s, "growth centers" sprang up all over the
United States in imitation of Esalen, featuring not only the journalisti-
cally sensational encounter marathons, Gestalt therapy groups, training in
meditation systems, lectures on mythology and Reichian psychotherapy,

but also providing a platform for teachers of Oriental acupuncture, muscle relaxation techniques, and a host of other approaches to what was called "psychophysical synthesis." Such centers soon provided platforms for other classical ways of healing: homeopathy, herbalism, chiropractic, Yogic therapy and Ayurvedic medicine—all systems that share at least a part of the holistic philosophy, and emphasize in curative terms, just as the purely psychological therapies did, the assumption of increased responsibility by the individual for his or her own well-being. The influence of Eastern philosophies and religions, stressing as they did not the worship of a single god but the emulation of all gods, reinforced the idea that holism meant not only the person in his entirety, but the place of the whole person as an integral part of the natural and man-made environment. Even semantically, the word "holism" was seen as related to the historical concepts of holiness, the worshipful notion that we are all intended to be whole and complete and bear a great part of the obligation to remain in that state.

Through both holistic streams of activity ran the theme of exploring the self-healing and self-regulating mechanisms that might be at work in the healthy personality. In a sense, illness and disease were seen as crises in healthy development, necessary, if painful, occurrences in the course of a normal life. Becoming and staying healthy was seen as more than mending broken bones or relieving chronic headaches; health became defined as not simply the absence of disease or disability, but the full expression of the human being's potential. A statement of René Dubos might have stood as the credo of both holistic medicine and holistic health:

> The components of the body-machine *react with* the environment, but living man *responds* to his environment. In fact, man's responses are not necessarily aimed at coping with his environment. They often correspond rather to an expressive behavior and involve using the environment for self-actualization. Health in the case of the human being means more than a state in which the organism has become physically suited to the surrounding physicochemical conditions through passive mechanisms; it demands that the personality be able to express itself creatively.

To a great extent, throughout the 1970s and the early 1980s, the holistic movement set up shop across the street from the medical establishment. With only 5 percent of the public budget of that establishment being spent on the promotion of health and the remainder devoted to disease management, many lay people were drawn to the alternatives offered under the banner of holism. "End of the line" patients, particularly those suffering from intractable conditions that had not responded to the exhaustive therapies of conventional medicine, sought out the other medicines: acupuncture instead of aspirin for arthritis, meditative practice or herbal teas in place of soporific drugs for insomnia, chiropractic rather than surgery for spinal disk debilitation. For some time it appeared that the holistic community would simply grow and expand along with the beleaguered traditional medical system, and eventually leave the populace of the twenty-first century with a choice between the two competing approaches to health care.

But the medical establishment had not been completely inert through the period in which holistic practice spread out from special centers to the community at large. A number of influential trends within conventional medicine itself were at work to revise, reform, and expand it. Establishment medicine, after all, has never existed in a vacuum, but has always been derived from and responsive to the cultures in which it operates. The past twenty-five years had seen not only the emergence of holistic perspectives in health and medicine, but a parallel change in consciousness about the human being's relationship to himself and his world. This raised issues of how we might survive with a knowledge that natural resources are finite, that we have been fouling the environment in fatal ways, that the dominant forms of social organization had separated the mass of people from control over their own lives, that certain identifiable groups of people, ranging from women to asbestos workers, had been denied the freedoms and securities of the majority of others, and that one could demand to have something direct to say about decisions that affect the person, whether it be the disposition of hazardous waste materials, ways to generate energy, methods by which food crops are disinfected, or even what might be done to us in the name of medicine.

These new awarenesses, and the consumer consciousness and community activism that resulted from them, were reflected in changes in conventional medicine, too. Despite the "disease orientation" of that medicine, there had historically been a clear appreciation that the prevention of illness and disease was an equally important task on the medical agenda. For example, the incontrovertible evidence that the dramatic decline in the death rate during the nineteenth and twentieth centuries, a decline primarily in deaths from infectious diseases, had occurred not through the curative techniques of formal medicine but through hygiene and environmental reform, was well understood by the medical establishment. And physicians were also well aware that in our own time, when the so-called "diseases of civilization"—chronic and degenerative diseases such as mental illness, cancer, stroke, cardiovascular disease, arthritis, cirrhosis, chronic bronchitis and emphysema—dominate the medical scene, their efforts to curb the spread of these conditions is as central to their concerns as treating such dysfunctions with biochemical and/or surgical procedures. The philosophy that "to cure is good, to prevent is better," has inspired vast amounts of research in preventive medicine and also the development of an expanded field called "social medicine" within medical education, a field that stresses the training of family physicians, internists, and pediatricians not only in the most advanced curative treatments, but in "nonmedical" skills that deal with environmental pollution, hazardous work settings, the dynamics of rural and urban community structure—all the nonclinical elements that bear on health.

Likewise, holistic medicine did not have a monopoly of interest in psychological factors. While the holistic and humanistic psychologists were seeking ways to heal the "mind-body split," as they called it, traditional medical education, too, was working on a closer integration of the psychosocial with the biomedical. The health care team expanded to include psychiatrists and psychologists, not as sources for secondary referral, but as primary members of the medical staff. Perhaps most dramatically, the teaching of skills in family therapy expanded enormously at every level of medical education, injecting into the worldview of health care practitioners the perspective of field and systems theory, so that they could see their patients not simply as isolated carriers of disease but as members of family and community systems which were as much a part of them as they were of those systems.

This is a particularly salient point of overlap with the holistic attitude. The holistic theorists, too, were and are profoundly influenced by the field theory of physics and the "open system" theory of biology, and in many ways these theories are variations on Smuts's original theory of holism. Moreover, the preoccupation of holistic-humanistic medicine with ancient Eastern systems is based, at least in part, on rediscovering within them the philosophical principle of the individual's identity with the natural world, his unquestioned place in the universe not as an isolated phenomenon but at one with his fellow beings and his cosmos.

Along with the evolutionary development of preventive medicine and the promotion of psychosocial issues to the front rank of concerns in conventional medicine, there were other subtle changes in medical education and service that were occurring as the holistic alternative was emerging. Another such change that paralleled the holistic perspective involved the matter of the patient's self-responsibility for his own health and his self-treatment of accidents and illness. The era we speak of, after all, was a time in which the pulls and tugs between the defined classes of society —the classical struggle between labor and management, liberals and conservatives, rich and poor—were giving way to new, self-defined groups insisting on what was sometimes called "participatory democracy." The demands for civil rights, for body rights in the form of protection from unsafe cars, for human rights in the form of sexual equality, for survival rights in the form of resistance to nuclear armaments—all these grand and sweeping and organized constituencies declared themselves. Through all of them ran the theme of autonomy and self-reliance for the individual and the community. Depending on one's orientation, these rebellions were seen either as aspects of narcissism and self-preoccupation, or as authentic populist, decentralist political and social action. Whatever the ultimate historical verdict may be on the vocal, energetic movements of the moment, their message and their energy affected every aspect of modern life, including conventional medicine.

So through the years, that medicine has become almost imperceptibly democratized. The concept of the "second opinion" became a commonplace; the physician lost at least a small part of his monopoly on expert knowledge as the new fields of physician assistants, nurse practitioners, and more sophisticated nutritionists (and old professions such as midwifery and "practical" nursing) expanded in numbers and importance; the admonitory rhetoric of "patient education," previously colored by scare warnings and flat injunctions, underwent a subtle change of tone, becoming more respectful of the intelligence of the layman and giving him facts and research data instead of simply coercing him to take care of himself; and, finally, much of what had become standard "medical expertise" was demystified as stethoscopes, blood pressure cuffs, and pregnancy test kits were marketed as domestic consumer items. Millions of people around the world began routinely to do for themselves many tasks previously performed *for* them by doctors and laboratories. A tacit declaration of health independence took effect, reflecting the widespread desire of individuals to reclaim responsibility and to resist the intimidation, excessive costs, and dehumanization that often resulted from depending on experts, be they carpenters, plumbers, or providers of health care. The inevitable extension of such individual self-management led, too, to the formation of decentralized small groups of persons who organized themselves around health issues ranging from weight control to cancer, from single parenting to Alzheimer's disease. The new patient education expanded to include self-education and mutual aid, even in the abstruse subject matter that has historically been the exclusive province of the medicine men.

While it appeared for some time that the analogous evolutions of the holistic community and the conventional medical establishment would go forward separately or in outright antagonism and competition, leaving the lay public to choose as best it could, clearly, traditional medicine had the edge. The medical schools, the hospitals, the pharmaceutical and health insurance companies, every level of government (and all the governmental money in support of medical care) were and are committed to the Western scientific medical system. Holistic health and medicine had existed only on the fringes of the medical establishment, almost as an underground network of practitioners, with techniques markedly different from those of traditional medicine. So if the two movements—the establishment and the antiestablishment that Ralph Waldo Emerson so presciently defined as a repeated phenomenon in every age—remained separate and at war, the holistic perspective was likely to be overwhelmed by the weight and might of consensual medical wisdom.

But such a prospect would not take into account the momentum of the inchoate, persistent demand of human beings to share in the knowledge and skills that might enable them to live full lives. What is more, the word-of-mouth testimony that confirms the empirical usefulness of remedies and procedures outside those of the scientific establishment cannot be quelled by even the most autocratic and arrogant institutions in a society. The urge to synthesize the best available information, the resistance to letting narrowly defined cartels of power become the final arbiters of such fundamental issues as health and medicine, are too pervasive to allow the new and the innovative or the old and abandoned ideas to be ignored or forbidden.

For the holistic alternative to be taken seriously, to evolve into a compatriot rather than a competitor of "regular" medicine, it required only the articulate voicing of the merits of unorthodoxy to challenge effectively the majority view of "proper" treatment.

In 1979 that voice was heard, and, of all places, it was given a platform in the *New England Journal of Medicine*. For it was in that most respected of establishment medical publications that a layman, the former editor of *Saturday Review,* Norman Cousins, wrote a report of his own recovery from a disease called ankylosing spondylitis, a degenerative condition that causes the connective tissue in the spine to disintegrate, a disease defined so flatly as progressive and incurable that specialists calculated Cousins's chances of recovery at about one in five hundred. The article in the *Journal* (which later became the best-selling book *Anatomy of an Illness as Perceived by the Patient)* was a simple, low-keyed, but eloquent description of how, with the full endorsement and cooperation of his physicians, Cousins took himself off the standard medications for ankylosing spondylitis (as many as twenty-six aspirin tablets and twelve phenylbutazone tablets every day) and substituted for that treatment massive doses of vitamin C (as much as twenty-five grams a day—or at least twenty-five times the so-called "recommended daily allowance") and an "emotional" cure consisting of watching funny movies and rereading his favorite comic literature. His "treatment modality" was, in other words, laughter and ascorbic acid—and this for a terrible, incurable condition. Cousins made a complete recovery in every sense of the word, restoring himself to a full professional life and the whole range of his active recreations: golf, tennis, horseback riding, and the vigorous playing of classical music on the piano.

Though he took great pains to caution his readers that his recovery through a self-designed treatment program could not be guaranteed to produce the same results for other patients suffering from the same disease, Cousins's detailed and enthusiastic description had profound effects on the attitudes of the lay public toward both the medical establishment and unconventional medical treatment. His carefully documented accounts of the part that his own emotions, attitudes, and behavior played in combatting his disease made manifest many of the principles that had lain silent in the writings of both traditional and unconventional medical people for years. Cousins's approach to his illness called up the homeostasis theory of Walter Cannon, the notion that it is "the wisdom of the body" to be able to restore balance when, for example, as in Cousins's case, a person was suffering from adrenal exhaustion. And his approach involved too, the ideas of Hans Selye, who had shown in his pioneering work on stress (he had been the first to apply the word to a physiological condition in 1936) that adrenal exhaustion could be caused by emotional tension, such as frustration or suppressed rage. Cousins's courageous strategy also suggested the work of Jerome Frank and René Dubos, who had repeatedly insisted and demonstrated that nonmedical techniques could be used to marshal the *vis medicatrix naturae,* the healing force of nature that had, in one form or another, been the underpinning of ancient systems as diverse as Hippocratic medicine and Oriental acupuncture. (Coincidentally, during the same period that *Anatomy of an Illness* was reaching such huge audiences, there was a sudden flood of new and more detailed reports of the synthesis of ancient and modern medical practice in China, Tibet, and Africa, demonstrating that around the world there was an increasing move toward integrating the honored medical traditions of the past with the miracles of the latest technological medicines.) Norman Cousins's wonderfully written account of his experience stands as an example of the fusion of the holistic and conventional perspectives. It had the effect of creating an armistice before the war, a signal to two potential foes that each might stand to gain more from détente, cooperation, and colleagueship than from allowing differences and disagreements to further alienate them from each other. The moment of exploring the idea of fusion had arrived.

It would be pleasant to report that the moment was seized by both camps, that the holistic critics of traditional medicine had dropped their wholesale indictment of synthetic medications and futuristic surgery, that they had ceased to speak so shrilly about self-responsibility for health that they rightly incurred the wrath of those who detected in such rhetoric the theme of "blaming the victim"—seeing the sick and disabled and even the accidentally wounded person as having caused his own distress. Or to report that, on the other hand, the philosophers and policymakers and teachers of traditional Western Medicine had, en masse, confessed their humility about the fixed laws of standardized physics, chemistry, anatomy, and physiology by acknowledging that factors other than the material and measurable findings of those sciences might be involved in the healing process; that they had become openly curious as to why acupuncture, homeopathy, chiropractic, and other unorthodox systems had simply not gone away after hundreds or thousands of years during which they had been "superseded" by scientific certainties; that the teaching and research institutions had invited practitioners of the other medicines to participate in joint research and tests. And it would be equally agreeable to report that both the unorthodox and the conventional practitioners of medicine had both become more sensitive to the fact that patterns of disease and illness are often deeply enmeshed in the reality of political, social, and economic repression of millions of people in the world, and that disputes over the efficacy of myrrh powder versus a corticosteroid ointment for poison ivy needed to be part of a larger effort to deliver *full* medical attention to disadvantaged people. Yes, it would be nice to report that this joining of ideas and therapies had taken place spontaneously, as both schools of medical thought became aware of their common purposes, and acknowledged that they might have even common scientific ground.

However, this did not happen, except in isolated instances. Acupuncture did begin to appear here and there in medical installations as a form of anesthesia, or even as an alternative to methadone in treating substance abuse; a number of primary care clinics staffed by both Eastern and Western physicians were established; more and more conventional health practitioners, as they themselves became exposed to the techniques of clinical biofeedback training and some of the older forms of self-regulation of internal functions such as blood pressure, heart rate, temperature, and breathing, began to refer patients to people and places where they might learn adjunctive ways to alleviate the conditions that were being treated with the usual medications or surgery; a number of postgraduate medical education programs in some hospitals, already committed to the more comprehensive, multidisciplinary training of resident physicians, provided at least some education for them in the unorthodox medicines, or allocated elective time in which they could acquire that training through independent study.

On the unorthodox side, though many physicians and other practitioners originally trained in conventional medicine began to identify themselves as "holistic" and even created the American Holistic Medical Association and other professional groups that mirror the entrenched, old-line medical organizations, the holistic medical community remains clearly set apart from the establishment. To a degree, the label of being "alternative" lost some of its competitive or ironic edge; some measure of dialogue is sustained, especially on such shared concerns as "stress management" and the significance of "lifestyle" on human health. Today holistic practitioners—perhaps because they are still the "outsiders"—make a more concerted effort to communicate, to exchange ideas, and to make clearer that they are not denying the breadth and depth of the achievements of conventional medical science.

But the peace treaty has not been signed. Each side makes little effort to tell the public that it sees signs of cooperation, or that they hope to combine forces in an organized way on behalf of that public. Most people, as patients, still visit their regular doctors, and although patients may repeat some of the usual criticism of conventional medicine—its cost, its impersonal style, its treatment of people as walking machines—they see practitioners of the other medicines only when all available conventional treatment has failed. And their guides to unorthodox practitioners are other lay persons who have somehow stumbled into the world of "different" medical practices.

Few spokespeople for either the conventional or the unorthodox viewpoints consider seriously any possible integration or synthesis of their work with that of "the other side." *Complementarity*—that great lesson of not just Taoist and Buddhist philosophy, but of modern wave-and-particle physics, of split-brain research, of confluent education, of environmental ecology—is not yet the spirit or goal, let alone the battle cry, of either camp.

This book can be seen as part of the effort to urge a stronger, deeper, and more sustained consideration of the possibility of that complementarity. The problems of the world, and of the health of the people in it, are too profound to permit the continuation of dichotomous thinking that makes knowledge of different forms of healing into the subject of political debate or professional defensiveness. Simply because iridology is a questionable form of diagnosis, and foot reflexology a debatable form of treatment for sinusitis, and because both are practiced outside the medical establishment, labeling them as a form of "madness," lumping them together with every other unorthodox medical treatment, and dismissing the lot as a regression to belief in magic and superstition is a tragedy. Similarly, it is too easy to join the attack on the style and environment of many modern medical institutions and enlarge the criticism of surgery and chemotherapy into a blanket disavowal of all that passes under the name of modern medicine. It is clear that within so-called "holistic medical practice" can be found perversions and the meretricious marketing of unorthodox ideas; similarly, there are examples of charlatanism and distortions in the practice of conventional medicine. Neither of these facts is a persuasive argument against attempts at cooperation and complementary action.

I believe that the beneficial aspects of unorthodox medicines are in conflict with "our" medicine only in that they spring from differing views of nature and its processes. Yet enlisting their effectiveness does not depend on abandoning prevailing ideas about the world, its laws, or the human bodies in it; acupuncture, homeopathy, and herbal cures are used regularly on animals about whose philosophy we can hardly be sure. Moreover, there continue to be regular "confirmations", in modern terms, of the knowledge, skills, and utility of the older therapies. An interesting example occurred when a special issue of the British medical journal *Lancet,* (Summer 1983) was published in honor of Swedish scientist U. S. Van Euler, the discoverer of a brain chemical known as substance P. This chemical has long been thought to be one of the keys to the transmission of pain via nerve fibers, and has led to a search for substances that act as antagonists to it. In *Lancet* one article was devoted to the action of capsaicin, the pungent, primary active agent in hot peppers such as cayenne. Scientists doing research in substance P found that capsaicin selectively stimulates and then blocks some nerve fibers that end in the skin and mucous membranes, and that these affected nerve fibers proved to be among those that contained substance P. The hot pepper chemical releases such substance P and leads to its depletion in the nerve fibers. Other evidence included the finding that the application of capsaicin to the appropriate nerve also depleted substance P in dental pulp, and as a result, in the words of the New York *Times*, "vindicates the empirical approach of our ancestors to toothache. . . . Now, as it has in other cases, science has come to the defense of folk medicine. . . ."

The New York *Times* reporter unwittingly exemplifies the condescension and provincialism of many modern scientists when he speaks of "vindication" and "coming to the defense" of a remedy that for centuries has been known as a potent treatment for toothache—and many other types of pain. The tone and semantics of the report highlight the fallacy that whatever is modern and current or new in science is accepted as if the sources were authoritative, and we must therefore be amazed that "old knowledge" can be correct and helpful. We can turn back to it now only because of recent "confirmation." Perhaps it would be wiser to see such events not as validations, confirmations, and defenses of the other medicines, but rather as *translations* of useful knowledge from one language to another.

Were we able to see all medical knowledge without the parochial vanity of modernism, we could also see the other medicines as potentially complementary and supplementary to other treatments in dealing with distressful symptoms. We need not be confined to *either* scientific medicine *or* the unconventional therapies, but are blessed with the opportunity to use *both* the relevant treatments of the ancients *and* the modern, *both* the East and West, *both* the rationalist *and* the empiricist, *both* the sophisticated *and* the primitive. (Some conventionally trained American physicians, for instance, regularly administer homeopathic *arnica* to calm the nerves and mitigate the pain of emergency patients as they are being taken to a hospital for "standard" surgery; in a less dramatic but more common way, some of the same physicians are teaching their patients adjunctive relaxation and breathing exercises drawn from Yogic therapy to accompany the regular dosage of the conventional, synthetic medications to maintain lowered blood pressure.)

I am convinced that in an era of increasing desire for the self-management of our lives, and in a time when the general process of education in our society is again making of the teacher the *educer* of the learning abilities of the student, the other medicines offer a thrilling and expansive means for amalgamating what Manfred Porkert has called the "pool of universal science." It seems to me that, as much as possible, everyone who is hurt or ill, diseased or distressed, should have the opportunity to benefit by not only what is called "the best and the latest," but by *all* the treatments that might relieve or heal him, especially when the additional, complementary therapies, such as those described in this book, are relatively inexpensive and require little complex technology. Whether that treatment is performed *on* his body or mind by someone called a practitioner, or if a doctor (NB, from *docere,* "to teach") is the person who teaches him things to do for himself, seems to me not half so important as the fact that possible help not be denied him.

I am hopeful that the sort of labels I have used—"holistic" and "conventional," for example,—will in time disappear, and that the bridge between the sharply outlined and well-defended estate of the conventional medical empire and the unfenced, sprawling territory of the unorthodox will be so busily traveled in the next few years that we will ultimately be speaking not of this or that kind of health, but only of health itself—and that we will be served and be serving ourselves with a medicine that is of all peoples and for all peoples.

Life is so made that opposites sway
about a trembling center of balance.
D. H. Lawrence
Morality and the Novel

2.
CONSTANCY
AND CHANGE:
The Experience of
Chinese Medicine

Whether as a traveler or in his own city, the Westerner is lured to China-town by food, festivals, and curios. Once there, the neighborhood invites walking, browsing, window shopping, not only for mementos designed for export uptown, but even for the cooking utensils and mysterious delicacies in the hardware stores and markets clearly established to serve the local residents. Where only Chinese is written or spoken, the visitor usually moves on, always aware that beneath the surface of the assimila-tionist shops and restaurants aimed at him, thousands of people are living in small apartments on the cramped streets and alleys, living in ways he knows are different from his own. He visualizes better and more exotic food than he has just eaten, a clatter of chopsticks handled with uncon-scious dexterity, singsong conversation and the round-cheeked faces of children eating in silence. The tourist knows, of course, that behind the doors may be adolescent boys dressed in the nylon windbreakers and running shoes his own children wear, and that they may be his children's classmates, but always, as he sees a bag-laden older Chinese woman shuffle toward a house entrance, he is reminded that the door she closes behind her shuts him out of another Chinese world he cannot even imag-ine. Behind the impenetrable language, the long coats and tightened shoes, the taut and ageless skin of faces that do not crinkle or sag quite the way his own face does, behind the facade of public, mercantile Chi-natown is the transplanted tradition of Chinese social life, and the tourist can only shrug mentally with resignation at the impossibility of seeing it.

Unless, of course, as I did one day some years ago, the visitor has an appointment in a home. My destination was not one of the small flats in a nineteenth-century building on New York's Pell or Mott streets. I was headed for one of the large, unrelievedly modern New York skyscraper apartment houses that have cropped up on the edges of Chinatown's crowded center. The men and women who crossed the plaza in front of the building with me were, for the most part, dressed as I was, though they were speaking Chinese. Once beyond the noise of the street, approaching the self-service elevators, I might have been in any apartment building in New York.

The seventh-floor apartment into which I was admitted was clearly that of a middle-class New York family. A television set sat at an angle in one corner of the living room, a basket of toys in another corner. The shadows of a few crayon marks still showed where they had been carefully washed off one wall. There were no rare Ming vases in the room, no jade dragons, no calligraphic banners, and no incense was burning.

The doctor I had come to see, John H. D. Shen, was distinctly Chinese, a tall, smiling man, well-dressed in the summer style of a sophisticated New Yorker: an ivory silk shirt with a dark blue figured tie; well cut, pleated, light gray flannel slacks; and finely polished black loafers. Apart from his throatily accented speech and long, calmly composed Oriental features, the only overtly Chinese object in the room was a flat embroidered pillow on the corner of his desk.

I had accompanied a friend to Dr. Shen's home, an American physician and patient of Dr. Shen, who had been treating my friend for a chronic and painful stomach spasm. My own request to Dr. Shen was only that I wanted a "check-up" and assessment of my physical condition. At the time, I had no physical symptoms. I had been under great strain, to be sure, having just left a career of over twenty-one years' duration and having also separated from my wife. When Dr. Shen, whom I had never met before, and who knew nothing about me except that I was a friend of one of his patients, asked me what was bothering me, I replied that I felt fine but merely wanted him to "check me over."

The Chinese physician uses no instruments to make any observations of sensory details. He is trained, in fact, to maintain an "appropriate" distance—three to four feet away from his patient—until as Dr. Shen did, he beckons his patient to a chair for a reading of the pulses. Next to the desk, on the doctor's left as he sat down, was a chair to which he directed me. He asked me to roll up my left sleeve, take off my watch, and rest my hand and wrist on the red, fringed pillow. In front of him was his own watch, a black-faced chronometer, which he had propped up by bending its stainless steel flexible band into an improvised easel.

My left arm lay along the edge of the desk, palm upward. Dr. Shen reached across the desk with his right hand and placed his index, middle, and ring fingers on my wrist, not quite parallel as in the reading of the single pulse in the Western style, but at slightly uneven points on my wrist. His fingers, I noticed, were warm and dry. Over the next forty-five minutes he looked at me only occasionally and briefly as he periodically shifted his fingers to other positions around the circle of my wrist. From time to time, he glanced at the face of his watch, but never for more than a few seconds. After about twenty minutes of "reading" the pulses on my left wrist, he indicated with a silent gesture that he now wanted to do the same on my right wrist, so I shifted slightly in my chair and laid my other arm on the red pillow. Dr. Shen again put three fingers on my wrist and repeated the procedure. During the entire time not a word was said by either of us.

In the Chinese system there are six pulses on each wrist, three "superficial" and three "deep." Each of these pulses is thought to reveal any fluctuation in the flow of energy in and between the ten internal "organs" —gallbladder, liver, lungs, colon, stomach, spleen, heart, small intestine, bladder, and kidney—and two "functions": circulation/sex and the "triple heater."

This is not to say that the Chinese idea of "energy imbalance" corresponds to the organic diseases of these viscera that are at the heart of modern Western diagnosis. In traditional Chinese medicine most ailments are chiefly attributed to what modern science calls "dyscrasia" (an abnormal state or disorder of the body) of the five basic elements of the universe—water, wood, fire, earth, and metal—as reflected in the human body. This same concept of dyscrasia was a feature of early Western medicine. Galen, the Greek physician who lived in Rome in the second century A.D., a man thought to be second in importance only to Hippocrates as a medical theorist, based his therapeutics on diagnosing a dyscrasia or abnormal mixture of the four cardinal body fluids, leading to his designation of the fundamental pathological typologies: choleric, melancholic, phlegmatic, or sanguine. Plato, too, some five hundred years before, had been quite definite on the subject of humoral imbalance:

> Now everyone can see whence diseases arise. There are four natures out of which the body is compacted, earth and fire and water and air, and the unnatural excess or defect of these, or the change of any of them from its own natural place into another, or—since there are more kinds than one of fire and of the other elements—the assumption by any of these of a wrong kind, or any similar irregularity, produces disorders and diseases; for when any of them is produced or changed in a manner contrary to nature, the parts which were previously cool grow warm, and those which were dry become moist, and the light becomes heavy, and the heavy light; all sorts of changes occur.

There are twenty-seven pulse qualities as described in a classical Chinese medical text, *Shang Han Tsa Ping Lun,* written in the second century A.D., so Dr. Shen was examining a potential total of 324 indications on my wrist. For ordinary diagnosis, eight primary indicators on each of the twelve pulses are usually sufficient, and it was these primary pulse qualities he had been feeling for: fast, slow, vast, weak, slippery, astringent, stretched, or tardy.

A fast pulse is one with more than five beats in one cycle of respiration; a slow pulse has strength but actually beats slowly—less than four beats in one cycle of respiration; a vast pulse feels like powerful, swollen river flow (one writer describes it as "coming like a flood, but is weak and long when it goes away"); a weak pulse, as in Western medicine is felt as insufficient and soft, and then almost disappearing when the fingers are pressed down; a slippery pulse feels superficial and volatile, like a bead of mercury in the palm; an astringent pulse is deep and strong; a stretched pulse is tight, but thin, and feels threadlike; a tardy pulse is irregular, often intermittently skipping a beat. The dozens of subtle changes are poetically described in the *Nei Ching* (as summarized in a paper by Lu Gwei-Djen and Joseph Needham):

> . . . sharp as a hook
> fine as a hair
> taut as a music string
> dead as a rock
> smooth as a flowing stream
> continuous like a string of pearls
> slightly indented in the middle
> the front crooked
>   and the back delayed
> soft and fluttering
>   like floating feathers
>   blown by the wind
> elastic like a bending pole
> taut as a bow when first bent
> following up delicately
>   like a cock treading ground
>   or lifting a foot
> sharp as a bird's beak
> like water dripping
>   through the roof
> resonant like a striking stone
> rapid as the edge of a knife
>   in cutting
> vibrating as when one stops the strings
>   of a musical instrument
> light as flicking the shin
>   with a plume
> arriving like a suspender hook
> multiple as the seeds
>   of a flower blossom
> like burning firewood
> like leaves scattering

like visiting strangers
like a dry mud-ball
like mixing lacquer
like spring water welling up
like sparse earth
like being stopped
  by a horizontal partition
like a suspender curtain
like a sword lying flat ready to be used
like a smooth pill
like glory . . .

In Western medicine the reading of the pulse is an equally basic procedure. The pulse at the wrist, or at the carotid artery on the throat just below the jaw, or just in front of the ear, is a direct measurement of the heartbeat, and the rate determines how hard the heart is working to pump blood, carrying vital oxygen through the body. Customarily, the practitioner reading a Western pulse feels the pulse for six seconds and multiplies by ten the number of beats felt, the so-called normal rate being between sixty and eighty beats each minute. The pulse diagnosis of the Chinese physician, on the other hand, often takes two hours, and proficiency in feeling for hundreds of possible qualities of the pulse is considered to be the highest talent of a doctor. The pulses are the sensitive signals not only of current illness but also the history and the future of the patient's health, revealing to the skilled Chinese practitioner data ranging from the eating habits of childhood to the prediction of the sex of an unborn child.

In fact, after completing my pulse readings, Dr. Shen's first diagnostic words, delivered both as a statement and a question, were, "You drank too many cold drinks when you were younger, right?" Right indeed. As a boy growing up in the Midwest, I had consumed gallons of the popular soft drinks of my day: sarsaparilla and root beer were my favorites, but I had also regularly drunk other flavors of the well-known Moxie beverages, as well as Vernors ginger ale, and, above all, "ice-cold Coca-Cola," all of which in the 1920s and '30s cost a nickel for an eight-ounce bottle. The sales to youngsters of these popular drinks were kept constant not only by sweetness and carbonation, but by contests in which we all collected bottle caps so that we might dig out the cork liners to reveal a letter printed underneath until we had amassed letters spelling "Coca-Cola." When we eventually managed to get all the letters, we received prizes like roller skates, baseball bats, or even money. The risk for us was scraped thumbs and broken finger nails; the result was, at least on my part, the consumption of at least one and as many as six bottles a day, a habit I carried through World War II and into my thirties.

How could Dr. Shen have known this so many years later? The deep "heart" pulse on the upper portion of my left wrist was "slow" and somewhat "slippery," he explained, and this indicated an accumulation of "cold around the heart." This frightening phrase, it turned out, was not meant to convey a picture of permanently frozen tissue near my *actual* heart, but rather an indication of an imbalance of "coldness" in the function of the entire meridian associated with the heart. The health of my heart, or its functioning to keep my body supplied with nourishment of blood and oxygen, was not impaired. I did not have a cardiovascular disease and needed no treatment, but I was being told that my early habits had recorded themselves in my body and that I should be aware of a need to continue to stimulate the flow of energy in that important meridian. "Coldness" in any organ or function is a signal, in Chinese diagnosis, of past, present, or potential "stagnation" of the energy flow of the meridian associated with the affected organ. In the case of the heart the blockage or stagnation might take the form of pain in the parts of the body along the route of the meridian, or a problem with a primary function of the meridian, the circulation of blood. Just as important, stagnation of *ch'i* in the heart meridian is traditionally associated with the "damping of the spirit."

Meridians are the pathways of the energy flow that is being measured in pulse diagnosis. The idea that there is a constant flow of energy *(ch'i* in Chinese, pronounced "chee") in the human body is the essence of Chinese medical theory.* In the earliest known text on the system, the *Nei Ching,* or *The Yellow Emperor's Classic of Internal Medicine,* believed to have been written during the reign of Emperor Huang-ti (2697–2596 B.C.), the principle of energy flow is at one point made the bedrock of all ensuing therapeutic methods:

> The root of the way of life, of birth and change is Ch'i (energy); the myriad things of heaven and earth all obey this law. Thus, Ch'i in the periphery envelops heaven and earth, Ch'i in the interior activates them. The source wherefrom the sun, moon, and stars derive their light; the thunder, rain, wind and clouds their being; the four seasons and the myriad things their birth, growth, gathering, and storing: all this is brought about by Ch'i. Man's possession of life is completely dependent upon this Ch'i.

Even this ancient text, however, is not the original source of the concept of *ch'i* as the universal life energy. In an even earlier text attributed to the founding sage of Taoism, Lao-tzu, though the reference is not so obviously medical, the acceptance of the universe as being in constant

---

* The oldest and most widely used method of Romanization of the Chinese language is the Wade-Giles system, first published in 1859. In recent years another method, pinyin, based on a Romanization developed by Soviet scholars, has become the dominant style used in the People's Republic of China. (It is that change that has given rise to such revisions as writing "Beijing" for the city previously known as "Peking.") Since most of the root documents of Chinese medicine were first translated into Western languages in the nineteenth century, the Chinese words in this book are Romanized in the older, Wade-Giles method.

flux, in alternating waves of *yin* and *yang* energy, is made the first principle of the good and healthy life. We are healthy, enlightened, wise, fulfilled, and prosperous to the degree that we accommodate to this flow in the universe, and to the degree that the corresponding flow of *ch'i* energy within us is in balance. What we call the indications of life in human beings—our breathing, talking, sleeping, eating, even our ability to think, read, and hear—all are the results of the flow of energy, energy we draw from the air around us and from the food we take into our bodies. Chinese medicine, like Taoism as a philosophy, is based on seeking an inner and outer balance of energy flow. Man is encouraged to follow a way of life that is modeled after nature's rhythms as the ancient Chinese observed them: the cycle of night and day, the circle of the seasons, the "shady side of a hill" (the literal translation of the components of the ideograph *yin)* and the "sunny side of the hill" (the literal translation of *yang),* and all the other patent contrasts in the universe: moon and sun, earth and heaven, motion and standstill, joy and sadness, reward and punishment, left and right, and so on. These opposite qualities, however, are not considered antagonistic. That *yin* is "negative" and *yang* "positive" was not extended to mean that *yin* is bad and *yang* good. Both qualities are considered to be ever present; neither ever exists in an *absolute* state. "Within *yin* there is contained *yang,* and within *yang* is contained *yin"* is the principle of the dual components of universal unity that is embodied in the symbol known as the T'ai Chi, or the Grand Ultimate. *Yang,* the active, light, masculine quality, and *yin,* the dark, feminine, passive component, interact constantly to create the whole world of forms—"the ten thousand things." The most evident example of this fusion of opposites is the human race itself: as a male, man belongs to *yang;* as a female, woman belongs to *yin.* Yet each, male and female, is born of the union of both primary elements, and thus both qualities are contained in both sexes. (A principle that is shared in the Western view of human beings, all of whom produce estrogen, the hormone secretion associated with, and dominant in, the female; and testosterone, the analogous hormone identified with maleness.)

The expression of the *yin-yang* flow colors all Chinese thought and action and the Tao is taught as the philosophical, physical, social, psychological, and even medical way that man might learn to be more than mere flotsam on the ebbing and flowing river of *yin* and *yang* forces. The doctrine of Tao offers man, through disciplines like meditation, massage, and exercises (physiotherapy), herbalism, and acupuncture, the means to achieve balance with nature and within himself. A balance so achieved is health, and any imbalance the sign of illness. This emphasis on the rhythmic accommodation to the highs and lows, the triumphs and failures in life may seem odd or curious to us—yet it is the standard of the medical system followed by one fourth of the world's population for the past three thousand years.

The quest for the perfect way to balance in the universe was not confined to medical terms and therapies. The idea of striving for balance defined the Chinese worldview, inspired Chinese art and poetry, and defined the ideal life-span for man and woman as one hundred years, for as the *Nei Ching* says, "those who have the true wisdom [that is, live in a balanced way] remain strong, while those who have no wisdom grow old and feeble." Longevity and health were considered identical, and both the literature and painting of ancient China reflect reverence for the elderly sage as a model of wisdom *and* radiant health.

Although the *yin-yang* principle of energy flow is pervasive in the culture of old China, it has been difficult for us in the West to respect it as a basis for medical practice. In the seventeenth century Jesuit missionaries sent to China to introduce Christian doctrine to the Orient brought back to Europe some dramatic stories of the medicine of the Chinese, but traveling and exchange between the two cultures was too limited at the time to lead to any thorough study by Western physicians. Occasional nineteenth-century converts to Chinese medical theory embraced the energy system enthusiastically. A doctor in South Carolina, for instance, reported in the *Boston Medical and Surgical Journal* of September 14, 1836, that "acupuncture owes its efficacy to the transmission of galvanic fluid. . . . It is not inconvenient. Every house can furnish needles. It is prompt and effectual. I have never failed to produce the desired effect, in appropriate cases, within the space of a quarter of an hour; and in such cases the relief was permanent."

A hundred years later Sir Thomas Lewis wrote in the *British Medical Journal* that he had discovered an "unknown nervous system" not related either to the sensory or the sympathetic nervous systems charted by Western scientists. His report of a network of "thin lines" of circulation of nervous activity received little attention, even though some of the basic texts of ancient Chinese medicine depicting a similar physiological structure had been translated and published in France just a few years before by the sinologist and diplomat Georges Soulié de Morant.

But despite these earlier Western flirtations with the concept of the flow of *ch'i*, we in the West have been reluctant to see energy flow as a basis for understanding health or illness. To us "energy" is a colloquial, imprecise word suggesting enthusiasm, physical or emotional stamina, the characteristic of an animated personality, the verve of someone exhibiting strength or purpose beyond the average. We see it as a concrete human characteristic only when instruments measure the calories of heat we consume or expend; we can imagine ourselves as air conditioners or furnaces because we are offered a calculation of BTUs as evidence that we generate or absorb heat. But we cannot usually accept that an organized, systematic flow of invisible "energy" courses through us in rhythmic patterns, along invisible rivers called meridians, and reflected in the qualities of pulsations of the arteries at our wrists. Indeed, this system hypothesized by the Chinese has never been verified in the same way that allows us to accept the palpable circulation of our blood or our lymphatic fluid. The channels through which those vital liquids course have been confirmed to our vision, our hearing, and our touch, while the supposed channels of *ch'i* are known to us only through the results we achieve by manipulating sensitive points on those channels with acupuncture needles or moxa (an herb ignited at selected points on the meridians), or our fingers as we press or pinch those critical points (acupressure). The *ch'i*, accepted by the Chinese as more universal and ubiquitous than air itself, remains, like electricity, visible to us primarily by its effects. This analogy may be more than metaphorical. Research in China, Great Britain, the United States, and the Soviet Union confirms that the sensitive acupuncture points specified in the ancient texts are functionally distinguishable from their neutral surroundings and possess an electrical potential higher than that of the surrounding tissues. It can be demonstrated, by means of a thermocouple, that there is an alteration of temperature at each point (a higher intensity of infrared radiation and of the absorption of oxygen).

It was the qualities of this invisible flow that Dr. Shen was examining as he palpated my pulses. In his mind each of the twelve pulses he read were merely the reflection of the energy activity in the ten visceral organs and two functions, and when he pronounced my heart as having stored cold, it was the result of his finding a "slow" heart pulse, a pulse with fewer than five beats to one cycle of respiration. So while it had seemed that he was merely "taking" my pulse rather elaborately, he was, in fact, watching the relationship between the number of pulse beats and the number of my inspirations and exhalations of air. If he was following the *Nei Ching* to the letter, he took as a norm of my pulsebeats one expiration and one inspiration of his own, during which time a so-called normal pulse should have pulsated four times. (Often the Chinese physician will feel his own pulse in order to compare it with the patient's.)

The possible 324 qualities of *ch'i* flow revealed by my wrists were only part of Dr. Shen's speculations. As a physician trained for over forty years in the Chinese system, he was considering many other of the "myriad things" before he announced his diagnosis: He knew, too, that the volume, strength, weakness, regularity, or interruptions in the rhythm of my pulses varied, depending on the time of day, wind activity, atmospheric temperature, the relative humidity, the season of the year, and the climate of New York City. (This breadth of possible influences is remarkably parallel to the idea of Hippocrates, who wrote that "in diseases there is less danger when the disease is more nearly related to the patient in respect of *physis* [the constitution of the patient], habit, age, and season, than when there is no such relationship".) His strategy was based on the dictum that the task of the physician is to see, to ask, to hear, and to feel. He had been paying attention as well to my voice when I first shook hands with him, and what I took to be his occasional glances at me were really careful assessments of my skin color, the clearness of my eyes, and my emotional state. Skin color, for instance, has a special significance in Chinese diagnosis. The classic texts specify that a number of combinations of certain colors and certain viscera, as the twelve organs were called, denote health and others denote sickness. The extent to which the correlation of pulse qualities and the tint of the complexion are significant is exemplified in one of many specific instructions in the *Nei Ching:* "When the pulses of the liver and the kidneys coincide and the related colors [of the skin] are azure and red, the corresponding disease has destructive and injurious power." (The Chinese, incidentally, have always thought of their own skin color as white.)

Though my pulses were the instruments of specific diagnosis for Dr. Shen, he was not only carefully observing my skin tone in relation to those pulses and listening to my voice for the sounds of illness, he was also watching me for signs of stress, and even taking account of my body smell as possible clues to my condition. (Anyone who has been near patients with tuberculosis, or a child with a high fever, has noticed the particular odor that accompanies bodily distress.) Chinese physicians use odors as an especially significant diagnostic tool. Again, a passage in the *Nei Ching* called "The Treatise on the Truth of the Golden Box" underscores the point: "Yellow is the color of the center; it pervades the spleen and lays open the mouth and retains the essential substances within the spleen. Its sickness is located at the root of the tongue; its taste is sweet; its kind [element] is earth; its animal is the ox; its grain is panicled millet; it conforms to the four seasons, and its star is Saturn. And thus it becomes known that the disease is located within the flesh; its sound is *Kung;* its number is five; and its smell is fragrant and sweet." This passage is parallel to others covering other considerations: the colors white, red, blue, and green in addition to yellow; the elements fire, wood, metal, and water as well as earth; the tastes sour, bitter, pungent, and salty besides sweet; and the smells putrid, rotten, scorched, and rancid as well as fragrant.

The scholar Manfred Porkert describes the theoretical foundations of Chinese medicine as a "system of correspondence." To emphasize the connections between man and his own body and between man and nature that must be in balance if the individual is to be optimally healthy, the "correspondences" he speaks of go beyond even the range of colors, sounds, tastes, elements, and smells. As the "Golden Box" passage revealed, the relationship of body parts to a time of day, a direction, a flavor, an emotion, another animal, a grain, and even a star or planet are all appropriate clues to the message given by the twelve pulses. The mystery of the interior condition and activity of the body may be determined by the connections between the patient and any or all of the corresponding aspects of nature. If a patient expresses hate or disgust for a particular season of the year, or a specific color, or fear or loathing of an animal, or a distaste for certain foods—all these lead the Chinese physician to suspect an imbalance of energy in the corresponding organ of the body, an imbalance that must result in illness, disease, or discomfort.

Dr. J. R. Worsley, who heads the College of Traditional Acupuncture in Leamington, England, and who is considered one of the foremost teachers of Chinese medicine in the world (graduates of his four-to-six-year training program, for example, were for a long time the only practitioners whose training was considered qualification for licensure in California), is fond of one of the classical interpretations of the flow of *ch'i* as the supplying of fuel for the internal society of the body. In this metaphor, inspired by suggestive texts like the *Nei Ching*, which is written in the prose of legends and myths, the heart is king of the body, the remaining organs are the king's ministers, each with specific responsibilities: The small intestines are like officials who are trusted with riches, and create changes of the physical substance (which Porkert interprets as "the organ that receives and assimilates the bulk of food; in other terms, in it the fine and the crude, the clear and the murky elements of food are separated and redistributed"); the spleen is seen as the "Official in Charge of Distribution, Transporter of Energy"; the stomach is spoken of as the "Official of Rotting and Ripening," culling essential nourishment, integrating it and passing on its strength; the lungs, the symbol of "jurisdiction and regulation" are described as the "prime minister," the official who receives the pure *ch'i* from the heavens; the large intestine is called the "Dust Bin Collector, the Drainer of the Dregs"; the kidneys are the "Storehouse of the Vital Essence, the Gateway to the Stomach"; the bladder is the official in charge of eliminating fluid waste; the liver functions as a "Military Leader," who excels in strategic planning; the gallbladder is the "Upright Official of Decision and Judgement." (All this again sounds quaint and colorful, but other Westerners, too, have described the inner organization of the human being in societal terms. Consider, for example, Lewis Mumford's description of the human brain as "a seat of government, a court of justice, a parliament, a market place, a police station, a telephone exchange, a temple, an art gallery, a library, an observatory, a central filing system, and a computer.")

Each of these organs corresponds to the fundamental elements of nature, the familiar world the ancient Chinese inhabited and observed, the world of wood, fire, earth, metal, and water, and it was the interaction of these five elements, seen as the seasons past, from which the Chinese developed their basic theory to explain the flow of *ch'i* energy in the human body. Of these elements, Chi Po, in the *Nei Ching*, says, "their changes, their increasing value, their increasing depreciation, serve to give knowledge of life and death," to which the Yellow Emperor replies, "In order to bring into harmony the human body, one takes as standard the laws of the four seasons and the Five Elements."

The law of the Five Elements, in turn, gave rise to another fundamental law, that of mother-child. Taking as a model the interaction of the basic elements of nature—the endless cycle of trees of *wood* producing *fire,* the decomposed ashes of *fire* creating *earth,* the *earth* begetting *metal, metal* forming in the beds of the rivers' *water, water* irrigating, feeding and supporting trees of *wood* and so on—the Chinese saw that the energy of the universe, the cosmic correspondence to the human body's energy, moved in a cyclical harmony. If the body is the human recapitulation of that cycle, then, the organs corresponding to the elements have the same mother-child relationship. The kidney/bladder (water) is mother to liver/gallbladder (wood), the liver/gallbladder is mother to the heart/small intestine (fire), the heart/small intestine mother to spleen/stomach (earth), the spleen/stomach mother to the lungs/large intestine (metal), the lungs/large intestine mother to the kidney/bladder (water), and so on. (The special functions of the heart constrictor and triple warmer are also associated with fire, and thus share the parentage of spleen/stomach.) If one applies therapy—acupuncture, moxibustion, or acupressure—to any of the meridians, the action will simultaneously affect the "child" of the target organ. If the energy of the kidneys, for example, is found deficient by pulse diagnosis and observation of the patient, according to the law of mother-child, stimulating the energy within the lungs (mother of kidneys) will automatically increase the energy received by the kidneys, children of the lungs. In addition to stimulating the lungs, however, the energy level of the liver must also be augmented, so that the liver (child of the kidneys) does not absorb the energy from the kidneys. Every organ is both mother and child, in other words, and it is fundamental to Chinese medicine that treatment takes into account these family connections. The mother-child law, as set down in the *Nei Ching,* is a direct injunction: "If a meridian is empty, stimulate its mother. If it is full, disperse the child."

With the techniques of stimulation (sometimes called "tonification" or "augmentation") of energy, and dispersal (the freeing of blocked or congested energy), Chinese medicine moves from theory to practical, direct therapy, for these techniques are the work accomplished by needles, moxa, or fingers on the critical points of the energy meridians.

After Dr. Shen made his first pronouncement about my history of drinking cold sodas, he sat back and smiled. "You know the problem, don't you?" "Why, no! I have no problem that I know of," I answered. He sat straight up, looked at me intently, and playfully wagging his finger, he said with a slight chuckle, "More meditation." The word "more" was somewhat surprising, since Dr. Shen could not have known that I meditated at all. For over a year prior to meeting him, I had, in fact, meditated every day for fifteen to thirty minutes, having taken up the practice in the belief that the calming effect of the discipline and the regular schedule of "doing what I was doing when I was doing it," to use one of Lawrence LeShan's descriptions of meditative practice, would help me cope with the many changes in my life with a greater sense of control and levelheadedness. In the few months before meeting Dr. Shen I had, however, been far from as regular in my meditating. "You need to get back to center," he went on, "need to be calm as you go on. No herbs, no needles —just more meditation."

This does not sound much like a prescription, perhaps, but as I mentioned before, the well-known techniques of using acupuncture needles and prescribing Oriental herbs are only two arms of Chinese medicine, physical therapy and meditation being just as important in the overall scheme. The increasingly practiced movement system, T'ai Chi Ch'uan, is an example of the fusion of these other two branches of Chinese medicine. In moving slowly through the prescribed 128 balletic positions, the T'ai Chi student is engaging both in exercise and meditation, for the regularized breathing and concentration that accompany the traditional movements is very much like the practice of seated meditation. (The Japanese Zen meditation system, similarly, includes *zazen* [meditation] in motion" as well as *zazen* practiced in the familiar fixed position.)

By prescribing meditation Dr. Shen was being true to the highest goals of Chinese medicine: the prevention of disease and the maintenance of good health. Some legends say that in ancient times the Chinese physician was paid only when his patients were well, and though he did treat them therapeutically when they fell ill, his primary and most valuable art was devoted to helping them avoid the need for curative or palliative needles. Taken in this light, Dr. Shen's instructions were serious and cautionary, warning me of the need to fortify myself against the negative stresses of my rather dramatic transitions. In his mind the trinity of my body, mind, and spirit showed the effects of lifelong habits, and verified that my subjective sense of being reasonably well and fully functional was correct—but that problems with my health lay ahead of me.

The Needling Medicine

One story about the origins of acupuncture describes the discovery of the meridians of energy as a by-product of war. Warriors injured by enemy arrows discovered that though they suffered pain from the arrowheads lodged in their bodies, they were simultaneously relieved of chronic conditions from which they had suffered before going into battle. From their descriptions it appears the diseases relieved by these punctures were what we now call arthritis, bursitis, tendinitis, and other afflictions of the musculoskeletal system. The legend holds that when reports of these paradoxical injury-cures reached the capitals of the warring states, the most advanced of the Taoist sages engaged in concerted meditations on their own bodies in an attempt to map the precise routes of the *ch'i* energy as it coursed through them.

Whatever the inspiration for plotting the routes of the meridians and the locations of the key points along them, reference to their existence is an integral part of the earliest known Chinese medical treatises.

Each of the twelve main meridians associated with the twelve organs has both a point of entry through which energy—either of dominantly *yin* or principally *yang* polarity—enters, and a point of exit through which it leaves after circulating along the meridian. The point of exit on one meridian is connected to the point of entry on another by a secondary channel, and the sequence of the energy flow is clearly defined. Although this flow is "endless in all living things" it begins, in the human body, in the Lung Meridian *(yin)*, which commences in the stomach, descends to the transverse colon, mounts up to the diaphragm, enters the lung, rising to its apex and after circling the clavicle (collarbone), it descends along the inside of the arm to the outside of the thumb. The Lung Meridian contains eleven points. The next meridian, the Large Intestine *(yang)* is an ascending one, running from the tip of the index finger to the base of the eye, and containing twenty points. Energy then descends once more on the Stomach Meridian *(yang)*, along a path running from the head to the foot, and forming a series of forty-five points. The next ascending flow of *ch'i* follows the Spleen Meridian *(yin)*, running from the foot to the chest, with a series of twenty-one points. The exit point of the Spleen Meridian is located on the tongue, from which energy moves to the descending Heart Meridian *(yin)*, with only nine points, ending once again at the side of the little finger. The Small Intestine Meridian *(yang)* then takes the energy from the hand back up to the head along a course containing nineteen points. At this point, the Bladder Meridian *(yang)*, with sixty-seven points on it, takes the flow on a descending path from head to foot, from which the circulation rises once more on the Kidney Meridian *(yin)* from the foot to the chest, with twenty-seven points.

Once again there is a descending flow, this time on the Heart Constrictor (a *yin* meridian, sometimes called the Pericardium), which courses from the chest back down to the hand, with nine points along its path. The next ascending flow rises on the Triple Heater, sometimes called the Triple Scorcher or Triple Warmer, a *yang* meridian, a path running from the hand to the head with a series of twenty-three points. A branch from the tip of the eyebrow to an entry point in the chest brings the Gallbladder Meridian *(yang)* into the sequence, with energy flowing once again downward from the chest to the foot, with forty-four points along the pathway. Finally, the flow rises once more from the foot to the chest along the *yang* Liver Meridian (fourteen points along it), ending near the entry point to the Lung Meridian, where the cycle begins again.

Eight months after my visit to Dr. Shen, I had my first experience of the way acupuncture works to manipulate the energy flow of the meridians. Suffering from an acute attack of sinusitis, so severe that my impeded breathing interfered even with sleep, I went once more to the apartment in Chinatown, this time accompanied by Dr. Leon Hammer, another American physician who had been studying in England with Dr. Worsley, and who was now spending two days a week working with Dr. Shen in his practice.

Again, Shen studied the pulses on both wrists. He then signaled that we should follow him to a treatment room in another apartment down the hall. In what must have previously been the living room, a number of examining tables, all covered with white linen sheets, were set up, each surrounded by tall folding screens. A small head pillow was placed at one end of every table. No other patients were being treated as I entered and took my obvious place lying on my back on one of the tables. Dr. Shen pointed to a box of tissues on a small table next to me, and then pulled out of a cabinet a box of needles which he unwrapped and opened.

The fear of needles is common, and the fact that a number of needles are used in standard acupuncture make the prospect of such treatment terrifying to many people. The actual risks, however, in such needling, are minimal. Dr. David Bresler, the director of the Pain Treatment Center at the UCLA Medical School, where acupuncture is used extensively, has reported that in over 3,000 instances in which perhaps as many as 500,000 needles have been employed, there has not been one instance of infection, nerve damage, or organ damage of any kind. Even more dramatically, at the Acupuncture Project of the Substance Abuse Division of Lincoln Medical and Mental Health Center in New York, up to 130 patients a day have been treated with needles for almost nine years with no incidence of side effects.

Needles are specifically forbidden in a number of situations: when the patient is suffering from severe hemorrhagic diseases, localized malignant tumors, overexertion, an overfull or empty stomach, acute exhaustion, any cardiac conditions, or in people with extremely sensitive constitutions. In addition, a number of points on the abdomen of pregnant women are strictly avoided.

Acupuncture needles vary in size from a fraction of an inch to seven inches long, plus the handle, and range in diameter from one seventeen-thousandth to one eighteen-thousandth of an inch. In ancient China needles were made of gold, silver, wood, bamboo, or bone; most needles in use today are made of stainless steel or copper, the needle most commonly used being the No. 32, one *tsun* (Chinese inch) in length. In addition to conventional straight needles, a so-called "staple" is also used, particularly when a person is being treated for obesity or impulse control problems such as cigarette smoking or other substance abuse. The staple is actually a small circular piece of metal with a tiny needle at one end, and is used only on an ear acupuncture point, where it is left in place for one or two weeks between treatments. Each needle costs from fifty cents to one dollar, and they can be used twenty or thirty times, sterilized with alcohol or steam prior to each use.

Dr. Shen explained that he would be using six straight needles and that four of the needles would be attached to an electrical instrument on the table with the box of tissues, a rectangular black generator that would emit a steady flow of nine volts of electricity and cause a consistent tingling sensation in the points in which those needles were inserted. He told me that all six needles would remain in place for about a half hour, after which he suggested that I should remain on the table to rest. "You may want to use these during the treatment," he said to Leon, pointing again to the Kleenex box.

He sterilized one needle and with his right hand inserted it at a point about midway in the center of my forehead in line with my nose at an angle of about fifteen degrees. The prick of the needle was about the same intensity as a mosquito bite, lasting for two or three seconds. This sharp feeling was quickly succeeded by a neutral sensation that I can only call highly focused pressure: It was not so much intense as it was heavy, and persistently present, comparable to the feeling of keeping the edge of one fingernail steadily on one given spot on the skin. The next needle Dr. Shen inserted above the first, again on the center vertical line up from the bridge of my nose, but this time at the edge of my hairline. The sensation was the same. Two more needles were inserted transversally, one on each side of my nose at its widest part. Finally, a needle was inserted at an angle of almost ninety degrees in the fleshy part of each of my hands just to the side of the crease formed by my thumb when it was pressed against the hand. (The points on my forehead lie on the Bladder Meridian, the points on the nose are on a branch of the Stomach Meridian and the points on my hands are important points on the Large Intestine Meridian.) To these two needles and the pair on the sides of my nose Dr. Shen attached the prongs of electrodes that were plugged into the electrical instrument. He read the voltage dial closely and then flicked the on-off switch. Instantly, I felt the vibration and tingle of the electricity, and almost as quickly I felt the stirring of mucus in my nose. After a few moments I had the feeling at all six points that the Chinese call *teh-chi,* a sensation of slight numbness, a near heaviness, and an alternating expansion and tightness in the areas around each needle. Dr. Shen seemed pleased when I reported this sensation, and he explained that to the Chinese physician this feeling is considered an essential indication that the treatment will be effective, representing as it does both the resistance and the acceptance of the needle into the body's tissue.

The *teh-chi* reactions slowly dissipated after about five minutes, and I felt the muscles of my legs and shoulders relax as I settled into the experience. Soon even the electrical tingle in my hands and face seemed milder, and I became more aware of the flow of mucus in my nose and sinuses than sensitive to the needles or electrical current. No more than ten minutes after Dr. Shen had flicked on the instrument, this flow of mucus in my nostrils became so active that I could feel it beginning to drip from my nose. I opened my eyes and asked Leon to help me by putting Kleenex under my nostrils. Within a few more minutes he was bustling to keep up with my needs, as more and more mucus drained out. I was doing nothing to force this active draining, not trying to blow my nose or snort. I felt as though the fluid was simply being released, not in the way it might have been if a powerful mechanical suction device were applied from the outside, but rather as if it were being liberated by some internal opening of a dam that had blocked the natural flow. As the time passed and I accepted this relief, I became aware that my whole body felt more relaxed and lighter. I turned my head slightly so I could study the way the needles had been inserted into my hands. It struck me that the whole procedure seemed totally natural; the connection between the six needles in my body and the relief I was feeling was clear to me. While I could not claim to feel the reordered, balanced flow of *ch'i* energy within my body, the obvious stirring and movement of my own bodily fluids while my body itself was so quiet and unmoving seemed to me a sign that "energy" was not merely an abstract notion describing an attitude, but had a palpable physical counterpart within me.

At Dr. Shen's suggestion, I had another treatment a week later for my sinusitis, exactly like the first in all essential details. By that time the congestion had been greatly relieved, so I did not experience the same rushing and clearing response, but once again I went through the cycle of *teh-chi,* followed by overall relaxation, and then a direct, local flow of the mucus that had accumulated in my sinuses and nose.

The introduction of electricity to acupuncture procedures is a very modern addition. Electricity can be used diagnostically, since it has been discovered that the traditional points on the meridians have as much as twenty times less electrical resistance than other places on the skin. An ohmmeter, therefore, can be used in conjunction with classical charts to locate the specific points where needles should be inserted. Or, as in my case, an electrical charge can be used to stimulate the needles once they are inserted in the body, replacing the traditional practice of "twisting" or half rotating the needles in a counterclockwise direction every two or three minutes.

The contemporary research that has introduced electropuncture to modern Chinese medicine has also discovered a great many new points along the meridians, some researchers now believing that there are as many as eight hundred. Most practitioners, however, use only about 100 to 150 of the classical 360 specified in the ancient texts.

In the West particularly, there has been an increasing use of ear acupuncture as a basic treatment. In the view of those who postulate *more* than the 360 classical body points, the ear itself is the site of over 200 acupuncture points, each of them having a specific relation to an organ or area of the body. Furthermore, the traditional map of the external ear has for centuries been considered to represent an inverted miniature of the human embryo within the womb, with the facial region located in the lobe, the head in the antitragus (the elevation above the lobe), and the remainder of the body folded in the curve of the fetal position, around the outer rim of the ear, including the spinal column as represented by the curved edge of the antihelix and concha.

Working from this representative map of the entire body, it is possible to treat a wide range of disorders working only with the points on the external ear. One of the most impressive and sustained examples of this approach is the Acupuncture Project in the Substance Abuse Division of Lincoln Medical and Mental Health Center in New York. There a team of acupuncturists, working with the medical director of the project, Dr. Michael Smith, are treating up to 130 patients daily, six days a week. The largest portion of the patient population are so-called "hard-core addicts," most of whom have at one time been involved in methadone maintenance programs or other more conventional approaches to the problem of addiction and withdrawal. The results of ear acupuncture in this large, friendly clinic have been dramatic, with approximately 90 percent relief of symptoms in acute withdrawal clients, and with 60 percent of the clients remaining drug- and alcohol-free for at least several months after a series of daily treatments. The acupuncture treatment is often combined with supportive psychosocial counseling, and as the patient population increases startlingly, physicians and other detoxification practitioners from all over the world are visiting and training at the South Bronx clinic. They are drawn to this unusual facility not only because of the obvious success of the treatment, but also because the procedures are safe and nonaddicting, treatment is rapid and inexpensive, and the clinic demonstrates movingly that a democratic, cheerful, and open clinic appears to enhance the social as well as the physical recovery of severely addicted patients.

Some Chinese physicians believe that when the meridians and points were first mapped, practitioners used *only* their fingers to manipulate the *ch'i* energy, and that needles were introduced later in an attempt to extend the effects of pressure. (Dr. Michael Smith is fond of saying, "The needles are for the therapist—to give him some evidence that he's doing something real or concrete; actually the touch and the human contact are the real treatment".) In any case, the use of fingers to manipulate the energy flow and relieve symptoms has endured through the centuries, and acupressure is a technique available to patient and physician alike for the temporary relief of distress, ranging from headache and muscle tension to arthritic pain and menstrual cramps.

Like the needles, the tips of the fingers can affect the flow of energy along the meridian pathways, stimulating it when there is blockage, dispersing it evenly when a meridian is "empty." The affects achieved are not as profound or enduring as those accomplished in a full needling session, but when done properly, the manipulation can provide a direct therapeutic benefit, especially for functional disturbances (such as my sinusitis), in the alleviation of pain and the reduction of muscular spasms.

Clearly, the breadth and depth of the history of Chinese medicine makes it impossible for any of us to become skilled practitioners without a great deal of training. But acupressure offers an immediate possibility for helping us to deal with the daily occurrences of discomfort or pain that do not require the more elaborate treatments of either Chinese or Western medicine. It is a simple, harmless, and in most cases, effective treatment. It is certainly no substitute for more advanced conventional or acupuncture therapy when a pain or disability persists. In that way acupressure is comparable to the improvised splint or tourniquet employed in emergency situations, a field expedient whose virtue is immediate, if temporary, relief of trauma. Though the points to be manipulated are the same as those used in complex needling procedures, and the theory behind the technique is the same ramified Chinese medical system originated by the ancients, it is an easy and congenial form of treatment for a layman to administer to himself or another. Remembering that the underlying concept of energy flow includes not only the inner activity of one's body, but, just as important, the impact of the outer environment, the practice of acupressure can be seen as the connection between the inner and outer forces that comprise the cosmos in which all of us live.

Until a few years ago even those Western physicians who were using acupuncture successfully were conservative in their estimates of its comprehensive possibilities. Some were even cautioning that acupuncture seemed an inappropriate treatment for systemic, inflammatory, autoimmune illness such as rheumatoid diseases. More recently, experimental acupuncture treatments with this order of diseases, including the recent epidemic of AIDS (Acquired Immune Deficiency Syndrome), are demonstrating encouraging, if tentative, results in the relief of the symptoms of fatigue, night sweats, weight loss, and even the level of "T-helper cells" that are associated with the disease. Acupuncturists are still cautious about the efficacy of needle treatment, pointing out that acupuncture is most often valuable in the early stages of illness, and may have little value in the treatment of secondary complications of AIDS such as Kaposi's sarcoma or pneumocystic pneumonia.

In the meantime, there is hardly a family in the United States that has not had a member or has not known a friend or acquaintance who has had some exposure to acupuncture or Chinese herbs. Particularly in the case of low back pain, cervical spine problems, bursitis, tendinitis, osteoarthritis, shoulder pain problems—in short, the whole range of musculoskeletal problems—it has become acceptable, if not common, for patients to be referred by their physicians to acupuncture treatment. Moreover, acupuncture is increasingly being used for muscle contraction distress, migraine and cluster headache, and a variety of neuralgic conditions related to nerve injury. And perhaps the most provocative spread of acupuncture is occurring in the field that is normally considered at least partly psychiatric in nature: the detoxification of drug- or alcohol-addicted patients, the treatment of nicotine addiction, and assistance in treating a broad spectrum of common psychological distress, including depression and chronic anxiety.

Even given this expansion in the range of conditions for which acupuncture is being used, most practitioners still believe that there are specific situations in which the standard Western approach is superior. This is particularly true in the case of infectious diseases and in instances where structural changes in the body such as fractures or tumors are involved. In these cases, acupuncture can and does relieve some of the accompanying pain, discomfort, and anxiety that are the common sequelae of such conditions, but the basic treatment of choice remains the medications and/or surgery of Western medicine. In the treatment of hypertension still another integration of the two systems can be achieved. Acupuncture is used on "depressing" points to restore overall energy imbalance in the body, and that treatment along with dietary salt restriction can decrease the amount of antihypertensive medication required for blood pressure control.

We are still in the early stages of that kind of complementarity and integration. Health care practitioners who are trained in Western medicine, if they are interested at all in Chinese medicine and its possible applications in their clinical practice, must, for the most part, seek training outside the established system of medical education. (Indeed, the audiences for extracurricular workshops and seminars on Chinese medicine which are being offered now all over the world are made up predominantly of health care professionals.) But where Chinese medicine *is* being used, and particularly where it is employed as an adjunctive companion to Western diagnosis and treatment, the benefits of needles, moxibustion, and finger pressure are too convincing for us to ignore Chinese therapeutics or to look on meridians, acupuncture points, and the flow of *ch'i* as amusing artifacts of a lost civilization. Those beneficial results compel us to open the Eastern portions of our minds to a worldview that does not, at heart, compete with our own, but only serves to expand and enlarge it, just as the concepts of gravity and electricity broadened our understanding of the nature of ourselves and the world around us. For as St. Thomas Aquinas said, "Nothing is contrary to the laws of nature, only to what we understand about the laws of nature."

3.
THE POISE OF THE SOUL:
Hindu Medicine and Yogic Therapy

My maternal grandmother, Delia Guttenberg, was born in 1875 in a house on East 139th Street in New York City. Her parents, Bertha and Mark, had been brought to America from Europe as children, having both been natives of Stuttgart, Germany. Nana, as I called her, clearly recalled that in her childhood the northern tip of Manhattan was still somewhat rural, and she insisted that as a little girl she had seen sheep grazing on the corner of what is now 96th Street and Park Avenue. But despite pastoral recollections, my grandmother and great-grandmother (whom I also knew) were the essence of urban sophistication. The family had lived in busy cities for several generations in Europe before immigrating, and the family traditions and beliefs were unmistakably cosmopolitan. Until she died in 1961, my grandmother, who under the more American alias of Delia G. Lane had worked in the 1920s and '30s for her friend Jack Strauss in his store called Macy's, was the most fashion-conscious woman I had ever known, and I was always convinced that her notion of New York was epitomized by having once been in the dining room of the old Waldorf-Astoria Hotel at the same time as Diamond Jim Brady rather than by a memory of farmland on what became the site of thirty-six-story apartment buildings.

My grandmother was also a hypochondriac. She fit perfectly the technical definition of that term: "a person with a morbid or excessive preoccupation with matters of health or illness." On hearing my first sneeze, she would lapse from her well-schooled English into the colloquial but urgent, "Are you getting a *Schnupfen* [cold], dear." Despite my denials she would watch me carefully for any other signal of an infection, and pressed cups of hot tea into my hands at any sign of minor illness. On occasion, of course, I did catch cold, and Nana was on hand with still another remedy. On one of my childhood trips to New York City from my home in Indiana, I not only caught cold but after a week was still afflicted with a stuffed nose that made breathing difficult and sleep almost impossible. My grandmother could not bear seeing me so discomforted, and after three days of observing this congestion, she took me into her kitchen and said she was going to teach me a way to relieve my distress.

She heated water and poured a cupful. Into the wide-mouthed tea-cup of water she added half a teaspoon of salt and one-eighth teaspoon of baking soda, both of which she stirred until they had dissolved in the water. She touched her finger to the water, and quickly transferred her finger to my nostril, just inside the tip of my nose. When I assured her it was not too hot, she marched me into the bathroom and positioned me at the sink. She instructed me to lean over, inhale a bit of the mixture through my nose, and while bent over the sink bowl, to take the water up my nostrils as slowly and steadily as I could. She cradled my head gently, urging me to relax and let the warm water mixture travel toward my throat without swallowing, so that I could spit the water out through my mouth. The first time I tried the procedure I gagged desperately and experienced the same panic that occurred when I accidentally swallowed water while swimming. I imagined that what was happening to me was much like drowning, and I coughed and gagged for several minutes after the first experiment. My grandmother cooed reassurances that everything would be all right, and if I relaxed and concentrated on the water flowing not toward my eyes or stomach, but along the path from my nostrils to my throat to my mouth, I could manage the inhalation of water without any difficulty, and I would clear my nasal passages in the process. Bolstered by her guarantees, I tried again and again to take in the water as she had directed. The fourth or fifth time I attempted this strange inhalation, I realized that it was getting easier and that, indeed, not only was I able to control the intake and outburst of water, but that the insides of my nostrils were tingling slightly with each nose gulp, and that air was also getting into my nose with less and less obstruction. With much encouragement and approval from Nana, I managed to finish off the whole cupful of water, salt, and soda, and though somewhat breathless, and rigid in my shoulder muscles at the end of the treatment, I was unquestionably better able to breathe, and the gentle tingle in my nose persisted each time I took a deep breath. The entire episode, what with my alternating resistance and cooperation, took almost a half hour, but even Nana's pronouncement that I was "a good sport" did little to relieve my tension. By supper time I realized that the remedy had worked. I was infinitely more comfortable in my breathing, and when I announced my relief, Nana reassured me that if I got stuffed up again, I could repeat the dramatic "drowning cure" as often as I wanted and that she would stand by to help me.

At the time, I drew no grand conclusions about my grandmother's homely, if eccentric, solution to the problem of clogged nasal passages. Apart from this saline solution, the only other health wisdom I recall learning from her was the slow sipping of blackberry brandy for an upset stomach and the virtue of chamomile tea as a relaxant before going to bed. Her own preoccupation with health took the more conventional form of constant visits to the doctor, who, regardless of his specialty (she never knew a woman doctor), was always described as a "top man." I can remember my father, who paid Nana's bills, being outraged at her relentless dependence on medical authorities and her equally unceasing complaints about her aches and pains. She tolerated discomfort badly, and though she outlived my father, surviving almost to her eighty-sixth birthday, she did so without ever developing an acceptance of even minuscule disturbances. She was, in short, not a model of the patient, enduring, and self-reliant nineteenth-century grandmother, and I never knew how she came by her knowledge of the magical teacup.

Nana's distance from any folk tradition, European or American, was not remarkable, considering her sophisticated city ways. What made the warm-water nose bath—a procedure I have continued to use, on occasion, with increasing ease throughout my life—at all significant to me was that I never encountered it in my research or study of any of the medical traditions to which she or her family might have been exposed. Instead, I met up with almost the precise description of what Nana taught me when I began to investigate the history of Hindu medicine and Yogic therapy.

In almost every text I consulted, I discovered an allusion to the ancient practice, still recommended, of lavages specifically designed for nasopharyngeal hygiene. Every Hindu medical book gives serious prominence to the causes of congestive phenomena, and not only are there dozens of therapeutic procedures for dealing with them, the emphasis on preventive hygiene to avoid the congestion of nasal mucosa includes many procedures similar to Nana's teacup remedy. There are two separate terms used to describe the recommended washing procedures: Traditionally, the *neti* procedure is a lavage intended to render the nasal mucosa tough and resistant to the frictional effects of dust and other particles; the *kapalabhati* lavage indicates the cleansing of the mucosa with water and forceful currents of air. The terms appear to have become confused through the centuries, however, and though the regular washing of the nose persists as a basic doctrine in Yogic therapy, the designations have changed. Thus, Nana's lesson is described as an "orthodox way of washing the nose," or *vyutrama kapalabhati,* and is prescribed as follows:

Water is taken in the hollow of the hand, and held over the upper lip, touching the nose. The soft palate is pulled down, as also the mandible (jaw-bone). This ensures a sloping of the floor of the nose so that the water, when sucked, will flow only along the floor and not irritate the olfactory nerve-terminals above. The water is sucked into the mouth thus, and thrown out. The process is repeated twice or thrice. It is best to bend the head a little forward and downwards while doing this.

While this particular description does not specify either the warmth of the water or the addition of any other substances, the use of "ordinary salt" and "bearably hot water" is generally recommended. No references to bicarbonate of soda appear in the Hindu texts, so we may assume by whatever lineage my grandmother assimilated the remedy, the baking soda was a European or American embellishment of the nose-clearing saline solution.

Kapalabhati is a Sanskrit word: *Kapala* means "cephalus," or "skull," and *bhati* means "light," or "luster," and the regular discipline of advanced Hatha Yoga includes a breathing exercise described by that one word. The exercise is one of hundreds of *kriyas,* procedures used either as expiatory rites or cleaning processes, that form the basic Yogic practice of *pranayama,* the rhythmic control of breath, and the so-called "fourth stage of Yoga."

Over the past twenty years the growth of interest in Yogic practice in the West has been phenomenal. One can find Yoga being taught not only on nationally syndicated television programs, but in the basements of churches of all denominations, or by tutors who will give Madame private lessons in her home, in the tradition of the language instructors of the 1920s. All over the United States people describe themselves as "doing" Yoga on a daily basis, having been exposed to lessons in college. The postures and movements taught in these classes have taken their place alongside aerobic dancing, jogging, weight training, Finnish saunas, and the Jacuzzi whirlpool or California hot tub as standard components of the fitness craze that has been spreading across the affluent Western world.

What is being taught, for the most part, is a portion of the basic (and lowest) form of Yogic discipline, the system known as Hatha Yoga. In Sanskrit the word *hatha* means "a force" or "a determined effort," and wherever it is used, the word "Yoga," which is derived from the Sanskrit root *yuj,* meaning "to join, or bind, attach, and yoke," means "to direct and concentrate one's attention on, to use or apply." "Yoga" also implies union or communion. In a book called *The Gita According to Gandhi,* (an interpretation by the great Indian political leader of the *Bhagavad Gita,* the most important authority on Yoga philosophy), the editor, Mahadev Desai, describes Yoga as

the yoking of all the powers of body, mind, and soul to God; it means the disciplining of the intellect, the mind, the emotions, the will which that Yoga presupposes; it means a poise of the soul which enables one to look at life in all its aspects evenly.

Yoga is one of the six orthodox systems of Indian philosophy, and we in the West must remember that in the Indian tradition philosophy and myth are not dead matter or amusing fictions, but are taken as living powers that shape the existence of the ordinary man and are reflected in the fine arts and architecture, the literature, the social organization, and, inevitably, the medicine of the entire Indian culture. Yoga, as one aspect of that pervasive worldview, was essentially systematized by a legendary figure known as Patanjali, who was believed to have lived in the third or second century B.C. His book of classical Yoga *sutras* ("aphorisms") contains in 185 terse passages the heart of Yogic teaching: Everything in the cosmos is permeated by the Supreme Universal Spirit (Paramatma or God), of which the individual human spirit (Jivatma) is also a part. Patanjali summarizes in his concise text the means by which the Jivatma can be bonded to or be in communion with Paramatma. That means, in its most general form, the practice of Yoga, and the one who follows the path of Yoga is a Yogi, or Yogin.

The practice described by Patanjali follows a hierarchical pattern of discipline. In its first stage, Yoga begins with sensory, physiological practices, primarily through the adoption of prescribed postures *(asanas)* and breathing exercises *(pranayamas).* In a sense, Hatha Yoga, which is sometimes known as the Yoga of Vitality, both embraces and is a part of other Yogic practice. In learning to do one of the hundreds of breath control exercises, for example, one must clearly use the mind as an instrument of concentration, and conversely, in order to meditate in one of the traditionally prescribed forms, one must relax the activity of the muscles of the body. But Patanjali was clear in giving Hatha Yoga a basic but lower place on the path to possible enlightenment; throughout his *Yoga Sutras* the highest goal is the spiritual communion of the higher Yogas.

Each Yoga system is named for its *kriyas,* or the dominant actions of the disciplinary system. Thus, the Yoga of intellectual study and introspective meditation is known as Jnana Yoga, or "union by knowledge," in which the intellect seeks to penetrate the ignorance that prevents man from seeing his True Self (Atman) and distinguishing that True Self from his own empirical ego, or personality.

Bhakti Yoga, "union by love and devotion," is a discipline of focused devotion to one revered entity, either one of the Hindu deities or the divine principle believed to be incarnated in one's *guru,* or master teacher. Bhakti practice includes a great deal of ritual observance and the singing of songs of praise. (Hindu teachers of Westerners often cite St. Francis of Assisi as an example of a Christian Bhakti.)

Karma Yoga is the discipline of selfless action and service, as epitomized in the life of Mahatma Gandhi. He exemplified the central principle of this form of Yogic dedication: the total disregard of possible benefit to oneself from the steady worldly work that is the vehicle of the devotional discipline.

The *Bhagavad Gita* says of Karma Yoga: "Never let the fruits of action be your motives; and never cease to work. Be not affected by success or failure. This equipoise is called Yoga."

Mantra Yoga, or "union by voice or sound," is the heart of one of the most popular Yogic disciplines exported to the West, the system of Transcendental Meditation, as expounded by Maharishi Mahesh Yogi. The motif of this discipline is the rhythmic repetition of specific sounds or chants *(mantras)*, influencing the consciousness, and thereby enhancing the control of bodily functions as well.

There are other variations of emphasis that characterize Yogic practice: Yantra Yoga ("union by vision or form"), in which colorful *mandalas* (symbols) or visualizations of the inner mind are used as devotional objects of contemplation; Laya and Kundalini ("union by arousal of latent psychic nerve-force"), in which the breathing and posturing techniques of Hatha Yoga are directed specifically to awaken the psychic energy believed to be coiled like a serpent below the base of the spine, and which is taken up the spine, passing through several power centers called *chakras* until the state of intuitive enlightenment *(samadhi)*, which is the highest goal of all Yoga, is achieved. Tantric Yoga ("union by harnessing sexual energy") is practiced mainly in northern India and Tibet and, though it is looked at with some measure of disdain by adherents of other Yogic disciplines, emphasizes control of the sexual energies and the actual or imaginative union of male and female (Yogi and Yogin) as the ultimate ritual.

It is generally understood, however, that any and all of these Yoga disciplines are servants of the highest goal, the practice of Raja Yoga, "union by mental mastery," described by Patanjali in these words: "From purification of the mind and body also ensue to the Yogi a complete predominance of the qualities of goodness, complacency, intentness, subjugation of the senses, and fitness for contemplation and comprehension of the soul as distinct from nature."

The ladder of forms which Yoga practice may take clearly culminates in what we would call a spiritual goal, the highest purpose of the discipline being the transcendence of the corporeal body and its senses, in the belief that "pure" human consciousness, already a part of the cosmos, can attain divine communion with Brahma, the Universal Spirit. Yet despite this end toward which the true student of Yoga works, the path begins with an understanding that the biological body must be brought under the control of the mind through the mind's capacities to exercise the intellect and the will. Even Patanjali recognizes the discipline of the body as a means to discover the soul, and he enumerates the stages through which the divine quest must be pursued, designating them as the "eight limbs" of Yoga:

1. *Yama,* the understanding of the universal moral commandments.
2. *Niyama,* or self-purification by discipline.
3. *Asana,* posture.
4. *Pranayama,* the rhythmic control of the breath.
5. *Pratyahara,* the withdrawal and emancipation of the mind from the domination of the senses and external objects.
6. *Dharana,* concentration.
7. *Dhyana,* meditation.
8. *Samadhi,* a state of superconsciousness achieved through profound meditation, in which the individual aspirant *(sadhaka)* becomes one with the object of his meditation—Paramatma, or the Universal Spirit.

Each of these stages requires the learning of purifying and reconditioning techniques involving the mind and the body. The crowning achievement of Yoga, *samadhi,* means "to put together as one whole," and is conceived of in Yoga philosophy as the inherent power of mind and body to achieve what we call homeostatic balance. In this respect the principle doctrine of Yogic therapy resembles both Oriental medicine, with its emphasis on balancing the energy, *ch'i,* and the homeopathic principle of disease as a distortion of the life-force. The Hindu and Chinese views extend even into cultural parallels. The Chinese concept of *yin* and *yang,* the nonantagonistic opposite forces in all of nature, is, in Hindu tradition, seen everywhere in the representation of the deities Shiva (the god entrusted with the task of destruction) and Shakti (the goddess of the active principle of creation) as lovers, symbolizing the contrasting principles of the Absolute, but a pair of cooperative opposites. So once again, the implied definition of health as balance, as the harmonizing of opposing forces in both man and nature, is the bedrock of a curative, preventive, and promotive medicine.

Yogic therapy is explicit. Its medical practices are not to be viewed merely as expedient stopgaps for the relief of an isolated pain in the finger or a recurrent headache. The specific therapies that have derived from Yogic knowledge attempt to deal not just with the obvious manifestations of disharmony in the patient, but with the entire profile of a human being as a creature living in a particular environment, with idiosyncratic habits; ingesting food of specific kinds; standing, sitting, and walking in a unique way; and almost above all, as a human being subject to conflicts and disturbances in his mind and in his transactions with others. Yogic therapy, therefore, addresses itself to a broad psychophysiological map of human nature which sees human beings on the one hand as possessing astonishing powers of self-healing and recovery and on the other hand as prey to continuing and powerful assaults on their integrated harmony— all stemming from the divine energies within, the Hindu pantheon of gods.

But the ideas of anatomy and physiology that sprang from Hindu philosophy and religion did not end with a divinization of the body. As in the Chinese system, in many of whose texts the organs of the body are seen as an assemblage of powerful forces such as kings and ministers, human organs and processes may be thought of metaphorically and named devotionally. Yet the physical reality of human existence is not ignored; it has been studied and codified to form a basis for therapeutics.

The foundation of the Hindu idea of the composition of the human body is at one with its worldview that *all* things in the universe are composed of five elements *(bhutas):* earth *(prthui),* water *(jala),* fire *(agni),* ether *(akasa),* and air *(vayu).* The pervasiveness of these elements means that the foods we eat, the air we breathe, the water we drink—all the nutrients of existence—are composed of the same elements, and this in-tertwined connection again reinforces the fundamental human belief that the human being is the microcosm within the macrocosm of the universe. All living things are seen as inextricably interrelated, giving rise to both the physical and philosophical theme of Hindu thought, "The One in the many, the many in the One."

As in the Chinese system that followed it, in which the law of the Five Elements—metal, earth, water, fire, and wood—governs the *yin-yang* cycle of creation and destruction, the five universal elements of Hindu thought must be brought into balance if one is to be healthy. Yogic prac-tice seeks to stabilize the psychophysiological processes; it does so by means of exercises and disciplines addressed to balancing the elements themselves. Traditional Hindu medicine carries the goal of balance and stability further by postulating that the five universal constituents, as contained in food, create the three bodily humors which manifest the cosmic energy of the elements: wind, bile, and phlegm are the three *doshas,* or somatic functions. In Hindu thought it is the balance or imbal-ance of these three constituents that reveals, on the physical plane, the relative health of all living organisms.

This fundamental view pervades not only Yogic practice, but also the form of medicine that evolves from Hindu philosophy and religion. That system is called Ayurveda (literally, "the science of living to a ripe age") and, like Oriental medicine, is formalized in texts written by early physi-cians, among whom the "Triad of the Ancients," Susruta, (5th century B.C.), Caraka (2nd century B.C.) and Vaghbata (625 A.D.) are the authors of the authoritative encyclopedias *(samhitas)* that are the bedrock of Ayurvedic practice.

In addition to the three basic humors which are seen as the governing processes of the body, Ayurveda defines the components of the body that are produced by the successive transformations of food as it is "cooked" by fires in the body: food juice *(rasa)*, blood *(rakta)*, flesh *(mainsa)*, fat *(medas)*, bone *(asthi)*, marrow *(majja)*, and semen *(sukra)*. The health of these seven components known as *dhatus*, are subject to the condition of the three humors—wind, bile, and phlegm. When one of these three *doshas* is "angry" or excited, it increases in proportion to the other humors and damages one or more of the seven *dhatus* (blood, flesh, fat, etc.) so that medical treatment must aim to restore the affected body substance and restore the balance of the *tridosha*, the collective name applied to the three humors. As Ayurvedic theory evolved through pre- and post-Christian centuries, (it is probably the oldest healing art in the world), the physician was transformed from a *bhisaj*, a mixture of respected priest, witch doctor, and magician, into the equivalent of a true and respected *vaidya*, a man of wisdom. Susruta described the ideal *vaidya* concisely in the opening of his book as a person who must dedicate himself "to cure the diseases of the sick, to protect the healthy, to prolong life." (This may be the earliest formal statement of the "holistic" principle in medicine, honoring as it does the preventive and promotive aspects of health care as well as the curative power of therapeutics.)

The relationships of the five *bhutas* to the universe was not as abstract as suggested by the philosophical principle of man as "the microcosm within the macrocosm." As in Chinese medicine the ancient texts were quite specific about parallels, designating even the vowels of speech, geographical directions, and planets that are related to the five basic elements. Earth *(prthvi)*, for example, corresponds to the vowel *a*, the eastern direction, and the planet Jupiter, while air *(vayu)*, is the element of the north, of Mercury, and the vowel *e*. These relationships are still used by indigenous healers in parts of India, where elaborate rituals are used in what we would call the style of sorcery to make diagnoses. The symbols of these correspondences are the healer's clues to the supernatural causes of disease and illness.

In another similarity to Chinese medicine, the key to diagnosis in Ayurveda is the reading of the radial pulse, which is considered the most accurate barometer of the air, fire, and water conditions in the patient. The Ayurvedic physician places his first three fingers over the pulse at the base of the thumb; with his index finger he is reading the pulse of the air principle, under the second finger the pulse of the fire principle, and under the third, the pulse of the water principle. Like his Chinese counterpart the trained Ayurvedic physician is feeling for combinations of rhythms and patterns of the pulses to determine the cause of the patient's distress—or as a guide to preventive or promotive measures the patient should take to preserve his health. Where the Chinese system stipulates 324 possible interpretations, the Sanskrit texts of Ayurveda record more than 600 different pulse combinations, which are thought to reflect accurately all the possible states of health and disease in man. The use of pulse diagnosis is again based on the philosophical and religious conviction that the patient and his world are inseparable, that both are composed of the same essential elements, and that if an imbalance is discovered in, say, the air principle, causing a patient to suffer from chronic fatigue or weakness, an herb or mineral or a specific food known also to contain the air principle is prescribed. All the medicines of Ayurveda are composed of natural elements. Even in ancient times the *vaidyas* were also pharmacists, gathering and preparing medicines in a prescribed way, expressing the appropriate respect for the substances they sought, uttering the suitable *mantras* (sounds or chants), and attempting to preserve an atmosphere of ritual purity so that the drugs they prepared would be unadulterated and effective. Susruta mentions over 700 medicinal herbs in his encyclopedia, and the introduction of drugs from western and central Asia has swelled the pharmacopoeia to the point where several thousand herbs and foods are employed in Ayurvedic medicine today.

This Ayurvedic medical practice survives today throughout urban as well as rural areas of India, though modern anthropologists consider it a hybridized version of the ancient system. Charles Leslie describes the contemporary medical system in modern India as a pluralistic amalgam of "(1) the Ayurvedic medicine of the Sanskrit classic texts; (2) Yunani medicine of the classic Arabic texts; (3) the syncretic medicine of the traditional culture, which evolved among learned practitioners from the thirteenth to the nineteenth centuries; (4) professionalized Ayurvedic and Yunani medicine, which has continued the syncretism of the past, transforming learned traditional-culture medicine by assimilating cosmopolitan medical knowledge and institutions; and (5) cosmopolitan medicine." Leslie also points out that "folk medicine," "popular-culture medicine," "homeopathic medicine," and what he calls "learned magico-religious curing" all appear in various regions of India today, and that, moreover, some of the systems overlap, with physicians trained primarily in one system using medications and procedures from other traditions. But the heart of Ayurvedic medicine—the belief that harmony is the hallmark of the healthy relationship of man to nature—continues in a modern version of the ancient system, based on vernacular translations of the old Sanskrit texts, creating a parallel and complementary medical establishment that operates alongside the "cosmopolitan" or Western system that grew up under the British.

Neither the traditional nor the modernized version of Ayurvedic medicine has traveled to the West in the way that Chinese medicine has spread. Instead, the medical components of Yogic practice have become part of the enlarging community of world medicines under the banner of "holistic health." In the United States, despite the longtime interest in "Yoga classes," the medical practice has not been popular. In 1906, for instance, the psychologist William James, despite his interest in and respect for Eastern thought, wrote a friend who had extolled the benefits of Yogic breathing:

> What strikes me first in it [the letter from James's friend, W. Lutos-lawski] is the evidence of improved moral "tone"—a calm, firm, sustained joyousness, hard to describe, and striking a new note in your epistles—which is already a convincing argument of the genuineness of the improvement wrought in you by Yoga practices. . . . I have . . . in the slightest possible way tried breathing exercises. These go so terribly against the grain with me, are extremely disagreeable, and even when tried this winter (somewhat perseveringly), to put myself to sleep, after lying awake at night, failed to have any soporific effect. . . . But your sober experience gives me new hopes. Your whole narrative suggests in me the wonder whether the Yoga discipline may not be, after all, in all its phases, simply a methodical way of *waking up deeper levels of will-power than are habitually used,* and thereby increasing the individual's vital tone and energy. I have no doubt whatever that most people live, whether physically, intellectually or morally, in a very restricted circle of their potential being. They *make use* of a very small portion of their possible consciousness, and of their soul's resources in general, much like a man who, out of his whole bodily organism, should get into a habit of using and moving only his little finger. . . . May the Yoga practices not be, after all, methods of getting at our deeper functional levels? . . . *You* have indubitably got at your own deeper levels by the Yoga methods. . . ."

This letter, with its mixed tones of personal frustration and open admiration, is at the core of the gradual infusion of Yogic practice into American culture during the past seventy-five years. For despite his own inability to make progress with Hatha Yoga, James at the same time laid down a principle that was to become the credo of the human potential movement of the 1960s, a movement which further popularized Yoga, for whether they knew James's letter or not, the leaders of the "consciousness revolution" were committed to the idea that there *are* ways a person might learn to reach "deeper levels" through disciplines of focused mental concentration and control. The central Yogic principle that integrated functioning *(samadhi),* even in the face of internal and external stimuli, can be achieved through the use of an inherent power of adaptation is the essence of the idea of self-regulation that lies behind not only modern Yogic practice, but other systems as well: biofeedback training, the relaxation response, progressive relaxation, the many approaches to health and cure that employ meditative exercises coupled with mental imagery. All these systems of health promotion and therapeutics are unabashedly based on a conviction that the "voluntary control of internal states" is possible, and they differ only in the mechanisms through which

they attempt to teach such control. The significance of the principle of
self-regulation, moreover, is not merely a matter of technique, but also
implies a profound change in the doctor-patient relationship, since the
emphasis is on the patient's developing *subjective* control without benefit
of drugs or instruments, and making the physician or other health care
provider primarily a teacher and guide and only secondarily a healer. Up
to this point, of course, the techniques are learned only rarely from doctors, since most methods of self-regulation are taught outside conventional medical settings: at weekend workshops, Yoga centers, "growth
center" programs, and in the offices of "holistic" practitioners, most of
whom are not physicians.

As far as such settings may be from ancient India, and despite their
concentration on mastering control of psychophysiological processes,
they teach a method that stems directly from the *Yoga Sutras* of Patanjali,
where so-called "physical" exercises like the *asanas* and *pranayamas* are
presented as the prelude to "higher" psychological processes calculated to
bring the yogi to the attainment of *samadhi.* It is almost as if the "lower"
exercises, found by our modern definitions to be health-promoting, are
minor benefits, only incidental to the spiritual goal. Whatever the significance of this hierarchy, the techniques of "lower" Yogic discipline have
universal implications for health.

The practices in Hatha Yoga that have most engaged the western
mind are the exercises known as *asanas* (postures), *mudras* (neuromuscular
locks), or "sealing postures," *bandhas* (contractions of organs or parts of
the body), and *pranayama* (the rhythmic control of the breath). None are
"exercises" as we generally use the term to describe muscle development
or increases in sheer strength. Yogic exercises, while performed in traditional and ritual ways, are calculated to create a homeostatic balance of all
the psychophysiological processes governed by the central nervous system, and are designed to include the control not only of the obvious and
gross neuromuscular and neurotendinous portions of the body, but also
the eyes and ears, and, to a certain extent, even the skin. They are based
on the belief that the inherent power of adaptation to both internal and
external stimuli is intended by nature to help the mind and body maintain a state of balance or to regain it quickly in the face of disturbing
factors.

This does not mean that Yogic discipline relies exclusively on exercises to deal with illness or dysfunction. The herbal remedies of
Ayurvedic medicine are used regularly by even the strictest Yogis, and the
postures and breathing control are used as adjunctive treatments, specific
asanas and *pranayama* exercises addressed to particular conditions. The
Yogic view, like that of homeopathy, sees acute symptoms as a sign that
the organism is *successfully* battling the disturbance, and believes that in
most cases the body can take care of itself, echoing Dr. Lewis Thomas's

well-known remark that "most things are better in the morning." But Yoga does not have a totally laissez-faire attitude, believing as it does that if the patient and/or his physician knows the specific remedy for an acute condition, that agent should be employed for the relief of pain or dysfunction.

It is quite another story with the Yogic attitude toward subacute or chronic conditions. In these cases the Yogic position is that the body is failing in its fight with disturbing factors and cannot recover until the inner power of adaptation and balance can be restored. This failure is thought to be caused by bad postural habits, deficiencies in or abuses of the diet, or "conflicts within," what we would call psychological or emotional distress. But even though these are seen as the major reasons for the loss of internal balance, yogis do not believe in merely palliative measures. One semantic interpretation of the word "Yoga" holds that it means "well-armored" or "well-prepared," and this has led to the holistic emphasis on developing and maintaining the inherent powers of the person rather than prescribing a patch-up curative technique.

To the Yogi the manifestations of the inherent power imbalance generally display themselves in two forms: (1) the faulty circulation of blood and lymphatic fluid, which leads to chronic congestion or stagnation of waste products in certain areas of the body, creating toxic effects in the body as a whole (recurring sinusitis would be one example), or (2) a faulty pattern of neuromuscular and neuroglandular reactions, such as occurs in chronic migraine pain, or thyroiditis. Yogic therapy has always seen that these two disease patterns are related: If a person is suffering from a respiratory ailment, the resulting congestion of mucus in the nose, bronchi, or lungs not only makes breathing difficult but affects the rest of the body as well, because the amount of nourishing oxygen carried by the blood is restricted, and without the normal flow of nutrients to cells, and the converse flow of waste away from that tissue, the entire organism is weakened. And, of course, the circle of distress always includes mental or psychological distress as well.

There is nothing exotic or occult about the Yogic model of disease, except the "imbalance of the life-force" as the diagnosis of all illness. In the Yogic vision, the whole person is thought to be sick or healthy, and both the treatment and prevention of disease is seen as an integrated matter. The body and the mind must both be involved if balance is to be restored or maintained, and the postures and breathing exercises of the Yogic tradition are addressed directly to integrating the inner power of adaptation. Therapeutically, Yogic practice prescribes a specific pattern of postures and breathing exercises for specific conditions, ranging from acidity to varicose veins and including the familiar range of arthritis, constipation, diabetes, hernia, ulcers, and so on. This same spectrum of possible disease dictates the hygienic and preventive assortment of exercises that are recommended. A Yogic therapist prescribes specific foods and herbs for a patient who simply wants to maintain health.

The fullness of Yogic therapy has yet to reach the Western world. We know relatively little about the herbal medicines of India and Tibet, and only a few of them are available outside their local regions. Similarly, though many variations of Indian cuisine have become popular, the Indian restaurant menu bears only a passing resemblance to the dietary regime that might be recommended by a traditional Yogic therapist. The portion of their practice that has established roots in the West concentrates rather on the postures and breathing exercises that have become a sort of alternative calisthenics for the health-and-fitness-conscious Westerner. In the process of being imported into the culture, the connections between the *asanas* and *pranayamas* and the classical Hindu conception of whole health have been largely lost, and the millions of people who "do" Yoga look to postures to enhance the suppleness of their bodies and to breathing as a means of relaxation.

The principle involved in both these Yogic practices is self-regulation, the mental control of physiological processes, and, in a sense, Yogic therapy is dedicated to the idea of "psychosomatic health," the converse of the Western theory that psychological processes can cause illness and disease.

Psychosomatic medicine, which in the Western world has become a medical specialty in itself, is the logical outgrowth of the marriage of the dominant strains of psychological and medical research of the late nineteenth century. The impact of the Freudian ideas of repression (the tendency to exclude from consciousness unpleasant or painful ideas) and the conversion syndrome (the psychoneurotic reaction to conflict in which the id and the superego requirements are satisfied by the conversion of a repressed wish into a painful or unpleasant physiological symptom) demonstrated all too convincingly that the human mind has a considerable, perhaps an almost infinite capacity to control not only the behavior of the personality, but the accompanying behavior of the nervous system as well. Freud's early work with the phenomenon of hysterical paralysis alone was dramatic proof of that power, and succeeding researchers only elaborated and confirmed the inextricable connection between mental states and the physiology of the body.

In the West the attention of both psychologists and physicians focused on such pathological patterns, and the emphasis in both medicine and psychotherapy was placed on curative techniques. In the early part of the twentieth century, as more and more physicians influenced by Freudian ideas emigrated to the United States, the organized study and teaching of psychosomatic medicine increased enormously. But it was not until 1939, not even fifty years ago, that there was sufficient activity in the field to justify a professional journal, and again it was focused on the pathological or negative aspects of the mind-body relationship. Despite the proliferation of interest in psychosomatics, the underlying assumption of Western medicine continued to be the belief that physiological processes were governed by the "autonomous" or "involuntary" component of the nervous system, which, by definition, operates outside voluntary controls. The performance by Yogis in India of such feats as stopping the heart, controlling bleeding, lowering the body's metabolism or modifying pain in any way were thought to be alterations explainable only by speculation about self-hypnosis or other trancelike conditions induced by a kind of hysterical mastery of psychological states, fit only for the pages of the *National Geographic,* where photographs of transfixed Yogis, staring directly at the noonday sun, were published alongside photographs of fakirs inducing cobras to rise sinuously out of baskets to the tune of native flutes. In the West the control of mental activity that creates physical effects is left, for the most part, to drugs and surgery that can, by intervention with the chemistry or the mechanics of the body, produce the changes that correct impaired functioning.

Mind and body are thus kept separate in the continuing unfolding of psychosomatic medicine, research centering on the brain as a biophysical organ, merely a part of the complex interaction of physiological and chemical networks in the human body. The effects of feelings like anger or fear are considered only in terms of harmful changes they precipitate in such processes as the flow of blood, the spurt of adrenaline, the tension of muscles, or the increase in the pumping of the heart. Psychosomatic medicine devotes itself, therefore, to finding the remedies for these inevitable hazards to health, ways of overcoming the automatic and uncontrolled responses of the body to stressful thoughts, feelings, and experience.

With the revival of interest in Yogic practice in the era of self-exploration launched by the human potential movement, the principle of possible self-regulation arose as a forceful challenge to the notion that human beings are incapable of the voluntary control of internal states. The "automatic" processes in the body were suddenly defined as at least partly controllable, and the *asanas* and *pranayamas* of Yoga were found to enable the student to begin to affect his own temperature, brain waves, blood pressure, heart rate, sweat gland activity, and even the electrical resistance of his skin, and thus, if any of these processes was associated with illness or disability, to participate directly in his own treatment.

In the West this principle of self-regulation has even led to the development of an "electronic Yoga"—clinical biofeedback training—in which the confirmation that inner "involuntary" processes can be brought under control is presented to the patient in the form of digital readouts of that activity during a time when the patient is being instructed in a series of breathing and/or visualization exercises that are strikingly similar to Yogic practice. In the most widely used practice a patient is attached via electrodes to an electromyographic instrument which records the extent of involuntary muscle activity at the site of the electrode. Under the guidance of a clinician, the patient engages in a series of deep-relaxation breathing exercises and simultaneously observes the changes that occur in his neuromuscular patterns. As he relaxes, or in more advanced training begins to visualize scenes or moods associated with tranquility and ease, he sees, in the same kind of illuminated digits he has grown accustomed to observing on his alarm clock, that the neuromuscular activity quiets down along with his thoughts. The feedback signals that educate the patient to what is occurring in his muscles may also be aural—a sustained tone, varying clicks or bleeps, or amplifications of his breathing or his heartbeat. Other visual data may include a flashing light, a moving needle, or oscillating pens on a graph. For example, if a person is attempting to learn how to control his heart rate, he may hear, when he is first attached to biofeedback equipment, a sound at a higher frequency when his heart rate increases and a lower tone when the rate decreases. In the introductory phase of biofeedback training this range of sounds is usually experienced as a random pattern that merely demonstrates the variability of the heart rate, or the presence of an irregular or elevated rate. This monitoring process simply sets up one phase of the mechanism: The patient is getting direct aural or visual signals about his inner processes.

The next aspect of the training is also primarily informative: The patient is asked to take note of whether there is a pattern to the thoughts that are occurring to him during either of the two patterns of his heartbeat, or whether he can affect the feedback tone by altering the physical position of his body in the chair. The goal quickly becomes obvious to the patient: to alter the tone of the feedback signal by changing the pattern of his mental activity or physical position. Since the tone is merely an information measure of the function being monitored, the result is that the patient is overtly controlling that function when he is in the biofeedback training setting. The remarkable spread of such training since the early 1960s is clearly the result of the success of the process. In fact, every physiological function that can be appropriately measured and "fed back" to people linked to biofeedback equipment—electroencephalographs for measuring brain wave activity, electrodermal meters for reflecting galvanic skin response, electrocardiographs that measure a whole range of heart functions, and thermal devices that measure peripheral skin temperature—all these physiological activities have been subject to learned control. Using such equipment, patients have been taught to control a whole spectrum of what have previously been labeled "involuntary functions" —reducing high blood pressure, regulating irregular heartbeats, increasing or decreasing blood flow to particular body parts—and to cure insomnia, eliminate or reduce the frequency of migraine headaches, etc.

The speed and precision with which information about internal activity is fed back to and used by a patient in biofeedback has not only legitimized the method as part of the standard armamentarium of medical therapies, it also has made for greater understanding. As Dr. Barbara Brown puts it: "If some medical researchers are now teaching hearts, or the minds of hearts, to reverse a pathological condition, then medicine must be learning that relationships between mind and body are more powerful than they once thought. The concept of 'psychosomatic' is generally accepted as indicating the mental origin of physical pathology; research into biofeedback is the first medically testable indication that the mind can relieve illnesses as well as create them." Thus has "electronic Yoga" added to the Western scientific map of the human condition the concept of "psychosomatic health" to complement the pathology-oriented principle of psychosomatic illness.

The connection between the techniques of Yogic therapy, with its unquestioning traditional reliance on subjective experience, and modern clinical biofeedback training, with its emphasis on objective confirmation of the internal processes of the body, stands as a model for the principle of integration of the old and the new, in this case the Eastern and the Western approaches to health. If nothing else, the contribution of Yogic tradition has been to revive interest in many systems dedicated to self-regulation—hypnosis, progressive relaxation, and guided imagery, as well as biofeedback training. The Yogic philosophy supports the idea that neither the curing of illness nor the promotion of well-being need be left exclusively in the hands of others. Westerners, who have found Yogic breathing, postures, and meditation congenial, even in the midst of high-speed technologized living, have discovered not only a greater connection between the functions of their minds and bodies in a physiological sense, but have begun to see that the integrated balance of mind, body, and spirit that is the keystone of the Yogic concept of enlightenment, is, in modern terms, the description of what we call health.

4.
"STRANGE, RARE, AND PECULIAR": The Practice of Homeopathy

"Do you prefer the ocean or the mountains?" "Do you have a violent temper?" "Are you generous with money?" "Do you have a sweet tooth?" "A good memory?" "If you had all the money you needed, where would you go for one week?" "Are you fastidious about housekeeping?" "Do you gulp or sip cold drinks?" "Do you sleep on your left side?" "What time of day do you feel best?" "What vegetables do you hate?" "Do loud noises bother you?"

Such questions may sound more like parts of a personality quiz, but they are, in fact, only a few of the dozens of matters probed by the homeopathic physician in the first encounter with a new patient. That exhaustive interview may last as long as two hours, as the homeopath seeks to develop a highly particularized and complete profile of the person who has consulted him.

As wide-ranging and free-form as the questions may seem, covering as they do an almost infinite variety of mental, emotional, and physical characteristics, they are being asked because the homeopathic physician follows a strict procedure which leads to his prescribing the *one* medicine the patient needs to relieve the stress.

Chief among these rules is the law of similars that gives homeopathy its fundamental slogan, *similia similibus curentur,* "like cures like." Though homeopathists generally deny that their system is a "philosophy," emphasizing that it is a carefully elaborated, therapeutic system designed to treat "one single, whole patient with one single, whole medicine," the principle that like cures like is at least the ideological touchstone of homeopathy. (The word itself comes from two Greek words, *homoios,* "like," and *pathos,* "suffering," underlining its distinction from allopathy, or the application of *opposites* to combat disease or illness.)

The law of similars is not new. Over twenty-three hundred years ago Hippocrates wrote, "Through the like, disease is produced, and through the application of the like, it is cured." The principle was echoed again in the writings of the fifteenth-century physician Paracelsus, who described the value of using similars in healing by writing, "You there bring together the same anatomy of the herbs and the same anatomy of the illness into one order. This simile gives you understanding of the way in which you shall heal." But the beginning of the complex, modern system of homeotherapeutics occurred only 175 years ago in the work of the physician and chemist Samuel Hahnemann, who expanded the law of similars into a systematic, empirical health practice which he labeled homeopathy.

Hahnemann, who had become disaffected with the practice of medicine, became a translator of scientific texts in order to support his family, and in the course of this work, translated a book by a man named William Cullen on the action of Peruvian bark, or cinchona, in treating malaria. Not at all satisfied with Cullen's explanation of the action of cinchona bark, (whose curative powers were attributed primarily to its "bitterness"), Hahnemann chose to test the substance on himself, taking a series of doses over several weeks' time. He describes the results in these words:

> I took by way of experiment, twice a day, four drachms of good China Cinchona. My feet, finger ends, etc., at first became cold; I grew languid and drowsy; then my heart began to palpitate, and my pulse grew hard and small; intolerable anxiety, trembling, prostration throughout all my limbs; then pulsation in the head, redness of my cheeks, thirst, and, in short, all these symptoms which are ordinarily characteristic of intermittent fever, made their appearance, one after the other, yet without the peculiar, chilly, shivering rigor.

> Briefly, even though symptoms which are a regular occurrence and especially characteristic—as the stupidity of the mind, the kind of rigidity of the limbs, but, above all, the numb, disagreeable sensation, which seems to have its seat in the periosteum, over every bone in the body—all these made their appearance. This paroxysm lasted two or three hours each time, and recurred if I repeated this dose, not otherwise; I discontinued it, and was in good health.

With the completion of the experiment on himself, the idea of homeopathy was born, though Hahnemann was far too well educated and cultivated to believe that he had alone discovered the law of similars. He was aware of the Hindu, Hebrew, Arabic, and Greek roots of the notion that "like cures like." Moreover, he was as much a chemist as a physician, and in the years immediately following his medical education at the University of Leipzig, he had published a series of books on medicine and chemistry, and his early work *The Apothecary's Lexicon* became a standard textbook, leading to his selection to standardize the German Pharmaco- poeia. And he was thoroughly familiar with the consensual medical prac- tice of the eighteenth- and nineteenth-century physicians, whose quite brutal treatment of most illnesses was founded on the belief that offend- ing humors, or fluids, were the causal agents of distress, and must be driven from the body by every possible means. Those means included not only cauterization, blistering, purging, and bleeding, but also the pre- scription of such a broad spectrum of drug mixtures that some remedies included as many as fifty different drug ingredients.

Hahnemann recognized clearly that by dosing himself with large quantities of cinchona he had suffered all the classical symptoms of ma- laria, the very disease for which Cullen had been describing the Peruvian bark as a remedy. Further experiments with other substances convinced Hahnemann that the principle of "like cures like" was valid, and from this overwhelming experience, he deduced homeopathy's basic principle: *A substance which produces symptoms in a healthy person cures those symptoms in a sick person.*

The distinction between the healthy person and the sick one empha- sizes the part played by symptoms, the signs exhibited by an organism in distress. Homeopathy sees those symptoms quite differently from con- ventional allopathic medicine. To the homeopath, human beings—all liv- ing organisms, in fact—are unceasingly reacting to the environment and attempting to ward off danger and repair damage. The homeopath consid- ers that this self-preserving and self-developing function is not the exclu- sive responsibility of the body, or even of the mind, but rather attribut- able to a life-force that permeates and governs the whole person. It is on this cornerstone assumption about the process of illness and health that homeopathy is based; homeopathy is a vitalistic system, one predicated on the belief in the ability of the organism to heal itself, and the system that sees symptoms, therefore, as evidence of the organism's reactive powers. Believing as they do that these reactive powers *always* strive for cure, for harmony in the functioning of the organism and for a healthy balance between the body and the environment, homeopathists define symptoms, therefore, not as part of the disease process but as the organ- ism's inchoate attempts to cure itself. The profile of these symptoms therefore must be as comprehensive as the physician and patient can create, for the body's reactive force attempts to deal with stress by pro- ducing a unique set of symptoms which are the homeopath's clues to the one drug that will help.

The consideration of symptoms, of course, is the core of all medical diagnosis. As the allopathic physician interviews and examines a patient, the doctor's mind is making a connection between the symptoms brought in by the patient and the diseases the doctor is trained to treat. As he discovers an elevated temperature or tenderness in one part of the body, the physician is attempting to discover not what is unique or unusual about such conditions in the patient, but what is general and common about them. His confidence in his suspected diagnosis increases with each detail he finds that corresponds to the usual pattern displayed by a certain bacterial or viral infection, or other pathogen, and each such narrowing detail is leading him to the prescription of a drug (usually synthetic) that is known to destroy the offending organism, a "contrary" substance that will weaken or kill the infection. It is as if his tunneled focus were concentrated on a disease entity occurring in a body that had almost no other activities surrounding it. (He is, of course, aware of possible side effects of the drug he will prescribe, and he will be careful to warn his patient that the medicine may cause drowsiness, or thirst, or flatulence, or fatigue, and so forth, but the implication is that these secondary biochemical reactions are "minor" by-products of the necessary assault the drug is carrying out against the primary target, the infection.)

In contrast, the homeopath, viewing the symptoms as a manifestation of the person's unitary vital force, is concerned with knowing, not more about the disease, but more about the person whose body is battling the disease. He believes it is the *person* who is sick, and the body is signaling through its troubling symptoms the efforts being made to recover. Hence the need for the penetrating questioning in the patient interview. If the homeopath is to find the one drug that will trigger the self-healing process, he must know much more than even a careful physical examination or laboratory test can reveal. He must know where the patient is in his development as a human being, what his state of mind may be, what changes are occurring in the patient's response to the stressors of life, how the patient sees himself in relation to work, the environment, other family members, and so on. In conventional medicine, information like this, when elicited at all, is considered to be the "psychosocial" component of the patient's condition, used primarily to identify psychopathology that may require treatment or that exacerbates the physical distress that brings the patient to the physician in the first place. Subjective data, to the allopath, is secondary in importance to the objective information to be gained from measuring the chemical composition of the blood and other bodily fluids, the analysis of tissue samples, the measurement of blood pressure, heart rate, brain waves—in short, knowledge of the physiological changes that occur in disease, not knowledge of the symptoms themselves.

The homeopath, on the other hand, is more concerned with subjective data, believing that pathological changes are *"the result of alteration in the vital principle, and not its cause."* To the homeopath the appearance of symptoms is chronologically prior to pathology, and consequently prior in importance. The homeopathic physician believes that ensuing pathological changes are always preceded by symptomatic changes, and that his mission is to attend to these *symptomatic* changes in order to prevent further pathological deterioration. His attention is given, therefore, to not just the "important" symptoms—the most obviously distressful complaints of the patients—but to as many of the surrounding details as he can observe or learn from the patient himself.

The diagnosis that flows from this minute attention to and respect for the patient's reports of his characteristics and symptoms is based clearly on Hahnemann's own experiment with cinchona. Following that experience, he and other physicians began to elaborate the principle through a process which came to be known as "provings." Small doses of animal, vegetable, and mineral substances were given to healthy people for a period of two weeks to two months, and the symptoms generated by these drugs were carefully recorded in the exact words of the experimenters. At his death in 1843 Hahnemann himself had carried out or supervised provings on ninety-nine such substances. By 1900 over six hundred other medicines had been added to the Pharmacopoeia. From this practice, over the past 175 years, a compendium has been amassed that describes the toxic, symptomatic affects of over two thousand substances, and the system of provings (from the German word *Prüfung,* "test" or "trial") continues to this day in the homeopathic community. As in the standard double-blind method used in conventional pharmacological investigation, about half the test group are used as "controls," being given an unmedicated placebo. The materials involved range, in the vegetable category, for instance, from simple common plants like onions and St.-John's-wort to rare species like Indian hemp and wild indigo; a vast array of minerals, including familiar ones like gold, copper, mercury, and sulphur, and less common varieties such as borax, cadmium, and nitric acid; among the animal substances employed, the common honeybee, toads, a variety of spiders, wasps, and even rattlesnakes provide the basic ingredients of the homeopathic remedies. (Incidentally, in all the years that provings had been the central part of homeopathic pharmacological research, there is no recorded instance of ongoing distress or eventual harm to the experimenter.)

From fifty to one hundred people are usually involved in provings of these substances. The results of their ingesting quantities of these toxic substances have been fastidiously recorded in their own language. The reference books containing these descriptions are the bedrock of homeopathic diagnosis, and it is not at all uncommon for a homeopath to consult such texts during the course of the intensive encounter with a patient, as he seeks to get the "drug picture" of the person he is treating.

Homeopaths are understandably insistent that their medicine is geared exclusively to *human* distress; experiments are never carried out on animals (though homeopathic remedies may be used to treat them) on the grounds that animals cannot report the nuances of mood changes and the varieties of sensation induced by toxic substances. Since Hahnemann's day the process of provings has concentrated methodically on developing careful records of human symptom patterns, since the homeopathic treatment is exclusively directed toward finding the *one* medicine that will cure the patient.

With almost two thousand reported symptom patterns to consider, it is no wonder that the range of questions which headed this chapter is typical of the interview with the homeopathic physician. In fact, the patient making his first visit to a homeopath will usually be given a pamphlet entitled *How To Report Symptoms* as he takes his seat in a busy waiting room. He is advised to describe, when he gets inside to see the doctor, not only what is bothering him, but how his troubles began, and the changes that have occurred since the onset of illness. Further, a complete history of previous illnesses and injuries is required, as well as a record of recent treatments. He is urged to describe so-called "nervous feelings" of every kind: "likes and dislikes, desires, fears, timidity, hurried feelings, lack of interest, persistent thoughts, discouragements, discontents, over-conscientiousness, whether critical, irritable, easily confused, if he suffers from aversion to business or work, absentmindedness, changeable mood, difficulty of concentration, dullness of mind, whether he is easily startled from sleep or when falling asleep, or from noise or being touched; whether he becomes annoyed by noise or talk of others or by children; whether easily affected by bad news; whether better or worse from mental exertion, or when occupied; whether sensitive to offense or contradiction." In sum, the "strange, rare, and peculiar symptoms" Hahnemann discovered to be so important in diagnosis.

As in Chinese medicine, and in the Hippocratic tradition of concern with environment, the patient is also asked in detail about the time of day, night, month, or season in which he is better or worse, and whether he is affected by different kinds of weather: cold, heat, dryness, oncoming storms, frost, cloudiness, seashore breezes, low or high altitudes, thunderstorms, and so on.

Homeopathy is intensely concerned with skin eruptions and discharges—their color, odor, whether thick or thin, gluey or sticky, whether they cause redness or burning, rawness or pain. Likewise, the excretions of urine and feces are important. Again the color, odor, appearance, quantity, frequency, and urgency of urination are critical data. With fecal matter, the color, odor, hardness, and dryness are to be reported in exact detail to the physician.

The breadth of the symptom profile is essential to proper homeopathic diagnosis. The words one uses to describe symptoms are, in an astonishing number of cases, the same language used over a hundred years ago—and probably throughout history—and to the degree that they match precisely the symptoms recorded by "provers," may lead the homeopath to his prescription.

For example, nineteenth-century provings of belladonna include symptoms described in such words as "pupils dilated; throat dried, as if glazed; hoarse, loss of voice, ocular illusions, spasms, delirium"—all symptoms that are close in every detail to those associated with, among other diseases, scarlet fever, victims of which present the physicians conditions of dilated pupils; violent congestion of blood to the head with a throbbing headache; high fever with hot, red skin; cerebral excitement; dryness of the mouth and throat; and muscular twitching. Belladonna, therefore, is the drug of choice for the homeopath whose patient exhibits that range of symptoms, carrying out Hahnemann's basic law of similars: A substance which produces symptoms in a healthy person cures those symptoms in a sick person. It is this law which gives homeopathy the basis for its classifications of disease. The usual disease categories are largely rejected, and the homeopathic physician, if pressed, will say only that the patient has a "nux vomica disease," or an "aconite disease," or an "arsenicum disease," and so on. Thus, the disease is named for its cure.

The use of the similar as a remedy is, despite its long history, the basis of one of the typical reservations one might have regarding homeopathy. The first-time patient of a homeopath can bolster his wavering confidence by reminding himself that in allopathic medicine, the vaccines that have become so generally accepted as effective are, after all, based on the same principle. The immunity against smallpox, for one, was used by Edward Jenner (a contemporary of Hahnemann's) and following the dramatic success of Jenner's use of similars a host of other immunizations were developed. Pasteur's vaccine against rabies, made from the dried spinal cords of rabbits who had died from rabies, was the crowning achievement of nineteenth-century medicine, and the tradition was carried on in this century with vaccines for yellow fever, plague, poliomyelitis, and the use of a wide range of pollen and house-dust extracts to reduce allergic sensitivity to these substances. And serum vaccinations are not the only instances in allopathic medicine that are based on the homeopathic principle of like curing like. The drug digitalis, for example, so widely used in both simple and compound medicines for treating heart conditions, is known clearly to create severe heart problems in large doses; Ritalin, often prescribed for so-called hyperactive children, is, in chemical reality, an amphetaminelike substance, and, of course, radiation therapy, used therapeutically in a treatment of cancer and other tumor diseases, is well known to cause those various diseases when given in toxic doses. If the patient of either the homeopath or the allopathic physician must seek explanations for the therapeutic actions of many drugs, he is left only with the insight of Paracelsus, who said in the sixteenth century, that "all things are poison, for there is nothing without poisonous qualities; it is only the dose which makes a thing a poison."

Clearly, the doses of the substances tested by provers are toxic, or they could not produce or ramify a collection of symptom profiles. What has come to be known in homeopathy as "the law of the minimum dose" derived quite logically from this "proving technique." When, after his own provings, he commenced to prescribe similars, Hahnemann quickly realized that the often violent reactions—what he called "primary symptoms"—to the substances were a result of the large dose, and he reduced his doses in order to moderate those reactions.

Even homeopathic physicians themselves (all of whom are trained first in conventional, allopathic medicine, pursuing homeopathy only after completing their regular education) do not attempt to offer a "scientific explanation" for the principle that governs homeopathic prescription: *The power of a remedy, selected on the basis of the law of similars, increases with dilution, and the greatest curative power is to be found in the small, infinitesimal dose.*

Homeopaths reinforce their belief in this principle by calling the process of sequential dilution used to manufacture their remedies "potentization," thus emphasizing their conviction that the more a substance is diluted, the more profoundly and longer it acts and the fewer doses are usually needed in treatment.

When we look at the way homeopathic substances are diluted in the manufacturing process, it is easy to see why allopaths are skeptical of their powers. One part of a substance (an animal, plant, mineral, or chemical element from the list of two thousand substances mentioned before) is diluted in nine parts of distilled water and alcohol. (In some cases where the substance is not soluble in water, it is first triturated, or ground, into a fine powder either in a mortar with the aid of a pestle, or by special machines designed to triturate large quantities.) This mixture is vigorously shaken or "succussed" at least forty times, after which nine parts are poured out and nine new parts of distilled water and alcohol are added, and again the mixture is vigorously shaken. The process may continue as often as desired, and the description of the potency of the remedy is based on the number of steps of dilution: 3x, 6x, 30x, 1000x and so on, up to 1,000,000x; the lower the number, the lower the potency. Homeopaths prescribe the low dilutions in the majority of acute cases and the higher potencies in treating chronic conditions.

This simple, standard process of manufacturing remedies has been at the heart of homeopathic practice since Hahnemann's day (although in his experiments he stopped at the 200x potentization) and it is this process, even more than the law of similars, that is still the most mystifying aspect of homeopathic practice. In conventional chemical analysis it is well established that beyond twenty-four dilutions, no trace of molecules of the original substance can remain. This is based on the discovery of a chemist named Amedeo Avogadro, a contemporary of Hahnemann's, who discovered that the number of molecules in one mole of any substance is 6.0253×10^{23}. In the light of the Avogadro constant, therefore, in any homeopathic dilution beyond 24x (which, in chemical terms is 10^{-24}), there are no measurable molecules of the original substance still present in the dilution. Yet over the past two hundred years, perhaps millions of patients have been helped with remedies prepared by this process and it seems clear that we must look elsewhere than the laws of conventional chemistry if we are to explain the power of such highly diluted microdoses.

Most homeopaths do not attempt such an explanation, except for contending, in the tradition of all vitalist philosophies, that the "essence" of a substance may be beyond conventional chemical verification, and, just as important, that the vital essence of the human organism, its power to heal itself, is comparably immeasurable. In the broadest sense, then, the potentized homeopathic remedy is seen as the catalyst that stimulates the healing powers of the patient. In our time this is, for many people, an inadequate explanation, for we have become insistent that everything in nature can be reduced to an analytic, scientific explanation, an explanation based on our accepted views of the physical and chemical laws that have thus far been codified. And this view prevails despite the fact that most conventional physicians do not know why most of their drugs work, as typified by one rarely candid passage in a standard medical textbook on pharmaceutical therapies, in which the authors confessed that "there are few drugs, if any, for which we know the basic mechanism of action."

As a result of not being able to explain the action of a remedy which, under conventional chemical analysis, contains nothing but "milk sugar" the skeptic can only attribute the effectiveness of the homeopathic microdose to the "placebo effect." The word "placebo" comes from a Latin verb meaning "I shall please." In a strict sense any remedy given as a placebo is an imitation medicine, an innocuous substance with no known chemical effects, given to a patient to please his expectation of getting a curative prescription from his physician. The placebo effect, then, describes the fact that simulated medicines, dressed up to look like real drugs, often work to cure illnesses, presumably because *belief* that a drug will help appears to be a necessary part of recovery.

Even in conventional medicine, however, the placebo is being given new and serious attention. Recent research is beginning to suggest that the placebo is more than a psychological prop, and while the way these pseudomedicines actually work within the body is not completely understood, there is some evidence that they activate the cerebral cortex, which, in turn, activates the endocrine system, and particularly the adrenal glands. Placebos, used in dozens of different illnesses ranging from allergies to Parkinson's disease, have been shown to be dramatically effective, especially when the relationship between patient and physician is characterized by deep trust and open communication, leading to the belief of some researchers that the doctor-patient relationship *itself* is the most powerful placebo of all.

But the belief in the effectiveness of a drug is not required for homeopathic remedies. A number of experiments have been carried out with patients who were overtly hostile to the principles of homeopathy but who nevertheless responded to homeopathic remedies in the same way as consistent users of homeopathy. Even more dramatic, homeopathic remedies are used extensively—and successfully—with both domestic farm animals and house pets, none of whom could be said to have "faith" in their doctors or in the power of any particular medication.

There is, of course, a great deal of current speculation that the placebo effect may have some basis in a measurable reality. The preoccupation with defining "energy" in human processes is one such speculative effort, and, inspired by the growing interest in Oriental energy-based medicine, many healing techniques have been and are being developed that unabashedly claim to work in ways that foster the use of inner energy, or the energy of the electrical field surrounding the body (see Chap. 6). "Energy," in that precise usage, does not appear extensively in homeopathic literature as a rationale for its effectiveness, but as I mentioned before, homeopathy is a vitalistic philosophy, and as a system of therapeutics is based on the belief in the innate healing power of all living organisms. Every medical theory in history has had to contend with this issue, and varying attitudes toward it are the points at which such theories diverge. So-called "scientific medicine," which has come to dominate the medical scene, has increasingly tended to reject the idea of the reactive and curative power of organisms. Whether it has been called the physis, the *vis medicatrix naturae,* the unitary vital force, *die natur,* or *anima sensitiva,* or any of the other terms depicting the inherent healing power, the concept has been more and more rejected by medical systems that have embraced the positivist, objective, "fact-oriented" stance of consensual physics and chemistry. Even the currently popular concession on the part of scientific physicians that the majority of common afflictions are "self-limiting" is based on seeing infection, inflammation, or other disorders as simply "dying out," without crediting any human power in their disappearance.

Homeopathy, on the other hand, has, from Hahnemann's day to the present, adopted the principle of the vital force as a cardinal doctrine, and the contrast between the allopathic and homeopathic physicians is nowhere clearer than on the issue of what can be known or done about fostering this power as part of curative treatment. In his book *Divided Legacy,* Harris Coulter, the most distinguished writer on homeopathy, clarifies the two positions:

> The Solidists [Coulter's term for the nineteenth-century school of allopathic physicians working in the tradition of the Scotsmen William Cullen and John Brown and the American Benjamin Rush] claimed that:
>
> 1) diseases are entities with knowable causes;
> 2) diseases can be classified with respect to these causes;

3) symptoms are significant as indications of cause; hence, those which yield more precise information about causes are more significant for therapeutic purposes than those more distantly related to the cause.

Hahnemann claimed that:

1) disease is a derangement of the vital force;
2) the internal cause of this derangement cannot be known;
3) diseases are not classifiable with respect to the internal cause;
4) diseases can be known only through their symptoms; hence, all symptoms are of equal importance.

The final point of Hahnemann's theory once again underscores the significance of the doctor-patient dialogue in homeopathy, with its universal emphasis on the subjective description of mental, physical, and emotional conditions, and the corollary of the principle of symptom-significance led Hahnemann to another basic doctrine that ranks with the law of similars and the law of minimum dose as a cornerstone of homeopathic practice: the law of the single remedy.

Allopathy, with its conviction that causes of disease are knowable, has evolved an ever enlarging pharmacopeia of "broad-spectrum" drugs, in a kind of massive attack on all fronts. Because homeopathy does not share the conviction that the cause of disease is knowable, it likewise does not believe in the scattershot prescription of multiple remedies. The homeopath, on the average, spends a great deal more time in interviewing the patient than his allopathic counterpart, attempting to establish a symptom profile so detailed that the *single disease* which the patient suffers from will reveal itself in sharp definition. A homeopath would never prescribe one drug for a stomachache, another for a headache, and a third for sinus congestion. He might openly acknowledge that all three conditions exist simultaneously, but the symptoms associated with all three are, to the homeopath, simply a key to the underlying disorder in the inner defensive and healing system of the person. It is to that comprehensive and unified disorder that the homeopath wishes to address the single remedy that, through the provings, has been found to be specifically curative.

The search for the single remedy informs everything the homeopath does from the moment he greets the patient. The exhaustive collection of information that follows the opening of the interview is guided by this quest, and it is through the finest detail that the narrowing choice of the correct remedy can be made. If a patient, for example, complains of cold symptoms, the homeopath will not assume that the patient is merely a victim of the viral infection that is "going around," or even that the symptoms arose simply because it is the "season" for increased incidence of colds. The homeopath will seek to discover whether the symptoms were brought on by exposure to dry, cold air, or damp, cold air or even warm, wet conditions. Moreover, he will want to know about variations in the symptoms: Does some relief occur in cold, open air or in warm, dry surroundings? Are the affected mucous membranes dry or draining, and if there is much discharge, is it watery or thick, and what is its color? As much attention is given to what, in the patient's body or environment, makes the condition better as is given to those factors which increase or worsen the symptom pattern. Many of the homeopathic texts to which the physician refers in trying to pinpoint the precise single remedy will literally list these exact conditions. For instance, in describing the symptoms of a cold, one patient will identify himself as "better" in open air, which suggests to the homeopath the possibility of aconite *(Aconitum napellus,* or monkshood), as a remedy, while another patient may be quite definite as to his suffering aggravation of the symptoms in open air, thereby leading the homeopath to consider dulcamara (bittersweet) as the remedy of choice. But the homeopath does not stop at discovering only one variable. For example, in this case, where both dulcamara and aconite are among the possibilities, look at the other differences between them as contained in Dr. M. L. Tyler's *Pointers to the Common Remedies:*

Aconite:
> sudden onset from exposure to cold; to cold, dry winds.
> *nose:* coryza dry, with headache, roaring in ears, fever, thirst, sleepnesses.
> checked coryzas, better open air, worst talking.

Dulcamara:
> colds from cold, wet weather and snow.
> from getting wet, or chilled when heated.
> worse sudden changes from hot to cold.
> dry coryza, sore throat, stiff neck.
> coryza worse in open air.

The consideration of aconite and dulcamara is, however, only part of the homeopath's concern if he is prescribing for a patient with cold symptoms. There are dozens of other remedies that have a successful history as relief, including *Allium cepa* (onion), *Antimonium tartaricum* (antimony), *Arsenicum album* (Arsenic oxide), *Belladonna* (deadly nightshade), *Bryonia alba* (wild hop), *Euphrasia* (eyebright), *Ferrum phosphoricum* (ferric phosphate), *Gelsemium sempervirens* (yellow jasmine), *Hepar sulphuris calcareum* (sulphuret of lime), *Kali bichromicum* (potassium bichromate), *Mercurius* (mercury), and *Natrum muriaticum* (common salt), *Nux vomica* (poison nut), and *Pulsatilla* (anemone).

The sensitivity of the homeopath must be of the order of the professional detective, or the investigative journalist. Despite the overt avoidance of psychological language or tactics (the homeopath never assumes the patient is "suppressing" feelings, or that the extreme disgust expressed about certain foods, animals, or weather is a "conversion syndrome"), the homeopath attends to the minute details of the symptoms that brought the patient to him, deeply aware through training that only through such fastidious listening and contemplation can the single correct remedy be identified. The range of questioning in the case of a person with cold symptoms is as elaborate as that used in interviewing someone with the symptoms of rheumatoid arthritis, the homeopathic physician being committed to the idea that if more than one remedy is prescribed, it remains uncertain which is effective. As Dana Ullman, a well-known teacher and writer about homeopathy, has written, the homeopath is unwavering in the pragmatic search for "the one deepest, most individualized, most all-encompassing remedy for each person."

Whether the final choice of remedy is correct is naturally determined by whether cure is effected. Despite the most assiduous interviewing, the homeopath and his patient may discover that the remedy prescribed does not relieve the symptoms. (If this is the case, no harm is done, however, since the patient has taken only microdoses and will not be affected with the symptoms caused by the quantities taken in the "proving" process.) The so-called "standard dosage" in acute ailments is two tablets of the 6x potency every two to four hours, but the interval between doses relates directly to the urgency of the situation, and in an acutely painful condition such as an earache, a dose every fifteen minutes is in order. If there is no relief within one hour, the wrong remedy has probably been selected, and the case needs to be reassessed.

Generally, the rule as to prescription of dosages is that the original dose should be continued until improvement begins, at which point the interval between doses is increased, and when improvement is well established, the remedy is discontinued. Prolonged use of a remedy beyond the time it is needed may cause what homeopaths call an "aggravation," that is, the patient commences to "prove" the remedy by displaying symptoms like the test subjects who first took the remedy to establish its characteristics.

In homeopathy, despite the emphasis on the significance of symptoms as clues to diagnosis and prescriptions, cure is not claimed merely at the disappearance of symptoms, but rather when the patient has achieved what George Vithoulkas, another currently influential teacher and practitioner of homeopathy, calls "the freedom of the individual to express fullness and creativity in life." (This statement is an interesting echo of one of the statements of René Dubos: "Health in the case of human beings means more than a state in which the organism has become physically suited to the surrounding physico-chemical conditions through passive mechanisms; it demands that the personality be able to express itself creatively.")

In homeopathy, however, there is an additional yardstick by which
at least physical cure is determined. The principle has come to be known
as "Hering's law," being named for the man who is considered the "father
of American homeopathy," Constantine Hering, who was born in Saxony
in 1800 and emigrated to the United States, where, in 1835, working with
Dr. Henry Detwiler, he established the first homeopathic school in Allentown, Pennsylvania. (In the early days of homeopathy most practitioners
were of German extraction and most teaching was done in German.) After
the close of the Allentown Academy in 1841, Hering obtained a charter
for the Hahnemann Medical College of Pennsylvania, in Philadelphia,
which remained throughout the nineteenth-century the center of homeopathic education in the United States, and in fact, the whole world.

In 1865 Hering published a paper entitled "Hahnemann's Three
Rules Concerning the Rank of Symptoms," in which he reexamined
Hahnemann's repeated charges that the abusive use of medicines in allopathy, even though it may occasionally and partially have relieved superficial symptoms, nevertheless had the cumulative effect of driving the disease inward and "deeper" into the body, resulting in the disease assuming
a chronic form. In his essay Hering reaffirmed this idea and pointed out
that with intensification of a disease process the symptoms themselves
move from the surface to the interior, from the extremities to the upper
part of the body, and from the less vital organs to the more vital. The
corollary of this principle—which it is easy to see is especially significant
to the homeopath observing his patient—gives the physician the measurements by which he can determine if the patient's health is improving
or deteriorating. In summary, Hering's law of cure holds that healing
progresses from the most profound parts of the organism (such as mental,
emotional, and psychological functions and the vital organs—the heart,
the kidneys, the liver, etc.) to the more superficial areas such as the skin,
muscles, tendons, and extremities. Likewise, the healing process moves
from the upper part of the body to the lower, and, finally, the healing of
symptoms takes place in reverse order of their appearance.

Hering's law is another central reason for the breadth and depth of
homeopathic interviewing, and is another explanation for the apparently
obsessive concern with "strange, rare, and peculiar" symptoms. The attempt to record precisely when and under what exact conditions the patient notices, for instance, that a rash on the arms or legs appeared during
a bout of influenza, is understandably important in homeopathic treatment, since the one affliction—the flu—is considered to be the deeper
illness, and the superficial symptom of a skin rash is seen as the attempt
of the body to throw off the *general* illness causing the flu. The progress of
the two sets of symptoms is followed closely by the homeopath and his
patient, and should the dermatitis clear up quickly while the flu symptoms continue, the patient is not considered to be healing appropriately.

Even more important, the hierarchy implied by Hering's law gives a clear view of the rank of the components of health: A person's overall state of health is defined primarily by his mental state, secondarily by his emotional state, and only thirdly by his physical state. This hierarchy is not applied rigidly in homeopathic diagnosis in treatment, but is used as a guideline, especially with patients displaying a variety of symptom patterns.

Hering's law of cure has been interpreted by some people to cause a kind of telescoped or condensed recovery, especially from minor ailments. I had a direct experience of this phenomenon when my wife and I both developed early flu symptoms. Both of us were first aware of a feeling of tiredness and tenderness in our whole bodies. Our heads and legs felt heavy, and over a twenty-four-hour period we had times when cold chills ran up and down our backs, no matter how warmly we dressed. Each of us had only a mild fever, and a headache that felt like a band around our heads. None of these symptoms were frightening or severe on the first day, and we felt neither totally ill nor really well. We knew from experience, however, that our symptoms were signaling the onset of influenza, and on examining several homeopathic remedy guides we discovered that our symptoms were precisely described under the heading of *Gelsemium sempervirens,* the homeopathic remedy prepared from yellow jasmine. We took two tablets of the 6x potency of this remedy on a four-hour schedule, beginning on a Tuesday morning. Neither of us was bedridden, but we tried to take things easy and move through the day as rhythmically as we could. We continued the remedy, and the symptoms lessened steadily during the first twenty-four hours of medication. On Wednesday morning we both awoke to find our most severe aches and pains almost gone, but as we continued with our dosage of gelsemium, and our bodies felt better, we were conscious of a tiredness and strain similar to the debilitation one feels after a fever has "broken." We were by no means ready to declare ourselves perfectly fit, but it was clear to both of us that we were not ill but convalescent. We continued on a schedule of reduced activities, and also decreased our intake of the remedy, stretching the dosage to every six hours. By Thursday morning we both felt sufficiently restored in energy and free enough from physical distress to stop the medication completely and resume our normal routine.

It was not merely the foreshortening of what had been usually a seven-to-ten-day affliction that impressed us. What we noticed in particular was that we experienced all our symptoms through the three-day period in a reduced intensity, and never felt "drugged" or logy. There were none of the changes in any of our normal bodily functions that often accompany a course of synthetic drugs: no dryness in the mouth, no gastric distress, no loss of appetite or changes in elimination. *Gelsemium sempervirens* in the 6x potency, like all homeopathic remedies, is made up in small white pellets no larger than half the size of a kernel of rice. They are taken on the tongue, without water, and melt almost instantly in the mouth like soft after-dinner mints, leaving a mildly sweet taste on the palate. Homeopaths insist on this form of ingestion, believing that the essence of the remedy reaches the bloodstream more quickly in this fashion and thus begins to take effect almost instantly. In the case of the gelsemium neither my wife nor I were aware of any special sensations as we took the remedy, but many people who take homeopathic remedies like arnica (the homeopathic remedy prepared from the *Arnica montana* plant, for overexertion of the muscles, or bruising injuries from blows or falls or sprains) or *Allium cepa* (onion, for damp-weather colds, or summer allergies causing streaming eyes and nose), report astonishingly quick effects from these remedies. Likewise, the homeopathic substances associated with the relief of medical emergencies like bee or insect stings *(Apis mellifica,* honeybee poison), shock or pain in eye injuries (aconite, monkshood), indigestion or belching *(Carbo vegetabilis,* vegetable charcoal), food poisoning *(Arsenicum album,* arsenic oxide), sudden fever or inflammation *(Belladonna,* deadly nightshade), fretfulness of teething pains in children *(Chamomilla,* chamomile), injuries to nerves or puncture wounds *(Hypericum perforatum,* St.-John's-wort), nausea and vomiting *(Ipecacuanha,* ipecac), overeating or bloated stomach *(Nux vomica,* poison nut), or itching skin eruptions *(Sulphur,* the element)—all these, among many other homeopathic "first aid" remedies, usually afford at least some immediate relief.

Though these remedies can be taken immediately after an accident or the onset of any symptoms, the ideal homeopathic prescription calls for taking a remedy with a "clean mouth," without *any* food or drink (except plain water) for fifteen minutes before or after taking the medicine. Other substances interfere with the action of homeopathic remedies, and it is commonly believed among homeopaths that coffee or other strong drinks are particularly likely to prevent the helpful action of the remedy. Likewise, the storage of homeopathic remedies is important. They should be kept in a cool, dark place (most remedies are packaged in nearly opaque dark brown glass bottles) and should not be kept near strong light or heat or substances which radiate pungent odors such as camphor, menthol, mothballs, carbolic soap, or perfumes. The homeopathic remedies themselves should never be handled, except when taking a prescribed dose, and should never be transferred to other containers, or ingested if they have accidentally fallen out of the bottle.

The tablets and pellets usually prescribed are not the only form in which homeopathic remedies are prepared. All the substances are also available in granule form (especially useful if the patient is unconscious) and many of the remedies are also manufactured as tinctures (alcoholic solutions) for external application. In the case of a sudden sharp blow to the wrist caused by a heavy window falling, one would immediately take four tablets of the 6x potency of arnica, and repeat that dose every two to four hours. In addition, a lotion could be prepared by dissolving one-half teaspoon of the tincture of arnica in one cup of clear water, the lotion then applied with a clean cloth to the bruised wrist.

The interval between doses is determined, of course, by the acuteness of the condition. While the every-two-to-four-hour prescription is the generally recommended schedule, the urgency of the situation may dictate more frequent dosages. In the case of an intensely painful earache, for instance, a dose of aconite or belladonna every fifteen minutes is not considered excessive, but if no relief whatever is experienced after an hour of such a routine, the assumption is that the wrong remedy has been chosen, and the remedy should be changed. Even in emergencies the homeopathic principle of idiosyncratic symptom patterns applies. An earache, for example, can occur after a chill or exposure to the cold, causing the ear to be red, hot, and painful, though the pain may be reduced by warm applications, either with a heating pad or a warm-water poultice. Such a profile is the classic "aconite earache." Still another earache, though also characterized by redness of the external ear, may be accompanied by severe, throbbing pains, and the ears have a "stopped up" feeling. The pain may be made *worse* from warmth of any kind. If, in addition to these symptoms, the patient is more uncomfortable in the evening and at night, and craves fresh air, the pattern calls for pulsatilla, the anemone. In each case the dose may be the same, and the switch from one remedy to the other, as well as the size of the dose, is completely harmless. (All homeopathic remedies are harmless, and even the swallowing of an entire vial of 125 of the 6x potency of any remedy would cause no ill effects. Nevertheless, homeopaths, like all other physicians, insist that remedies be kept out of the reach of children.)

The foregoing represents a summary of the main principles and techniques of so-called "classical" homeopathy, a practice dominated by allegiance to three historical principles: the law of similars, the law of the minimum dose, and Hering's law of cure.

Currently, however, there is a major force emerging in homeopathy that departs markedly from the classical approach. Referred to by many as the "pluralists," this school of thought is led by French homeopathic physicians who are beginning to teach and have influence not only in their own country, but in India, Germany, Spain, Canada, Mexico, and the United States.

It is fairly clear why the French are in the vanguard of the revisionist movement. In 1965 the French Government "officialized" homeopathy by admitting homeopathic remedies into the standard Pharmacopoeia published and monitored by the Ministry of Health. Visits to homeopathic physicians (there are virtually no lay homeopathists in France) are fully covered by national and private insurance plans, as are the costs of homeopathic prescriptions, and there are now about eighteen thousand pharmacies in France carrying homeopathic preparations. It has been estimated that about 16 percent of the French population occasionally or regularly use homeopathy. The leading French homeopathic pharmaceutical house, Laboratoires Boiron, with headquarters in Lyons (which is probably also the world's largest manufacturer and distributor of homeopathic remedies, exporting its medications to dozens of countries throughout the world), has undertaken a massive educational, publishing, and research program, seeking to spread the pluralist approach to the practice of homeopathy.

The French pluralist approach differs from the classical style primarily in its deemphasis of the treatment of mental and emotional symptoms and its virtually total disdain for the claim that homeopathic treatment affects the "vital living force." Homeopathy, these pluralists insist, is simply the outgrowth of the scientific, experimental medicine devised by Hahnemann and revised by him periodically in the light of continuing experiments over almost fifty years. The pluralist interview and diagnosis are very much like the classical allopathic doctor-patient encounter, concentrating almost exclusively on the physical examination and objectively observed conditions, seeking to arrive at a differential conclusion in almost the same fashion as conventional doctors. Once that diagnosis is made, however, the treatment is usually homeopathic, although in another departure from the classical approach, the pluralist may prescribe many more than the one remedy which is the hallmark of classical homeopathic treatment. Moreover, the French pluralists not only make no objection to the use of allopathic medications, but often employ them along with homeopathic remedies. Nor do the pluralists insist on the injunction against drinking coffee or taking medicines only with a "clean mouth," claiming that other substances cannot interfere with the effect of homeopathic preparations which, they say, act on a "different level."

To some the pluralist approach seems not to be homeopathy at all, but simply good allopathic medical practice that substitutes standard homeopathic remedies for the broad-spectrum, synthetic medications of establishment medicine. This criticism is reinforced by the pluralists' abrupt dismissal of the vitalistic philosophy that inspires classical practice, a philosophy that deals with the subtleties and nuances of human spirit and attitudes and emotional states. To the pluralist, as to the allopathic skeptics about homeopathy, that sort of consideration in medical practice introduces metaphysics into science, which they find intolerable. A pluralist homeopathist might say to a classical colleague, "You may believe, if you wish, that the effectiveness of homeopathic remedies—'like cures like'—is a metaphysical law, but you cannot work with that law, and must, instead, be a well-trained, scientifically oriented physician if you are to treat your patients successfully. You are dealing with a somatopsychic unity in human beings, not treating psychosomatic illness."

In this spirit of "scientific" homeopathy a large amount of research has already been launched in France and elsewhere in Europe, and the forceful proponents of pluralist homeopathy have also been the first in their field to convince some orthodox medical schools in France to include a homeopathic curriculum. Those who speak for this "other" homeopathy are impressively trained, intelligent, and vigorous people. They may appear almost missionary in their tone, close to scornful of those followers of Kent and Hering whom they consider "visionary," and too preoccupied with sheerly physical diagnosis to make their stand appealing to holistic practitioners, but they represent a lively and irrepressible force which, over the next few years of further research and practice, will doubtless have immense influence, not only among homeopaths, but also among orthodox physicians, who are likely to find the pragmatic French approach more attractive than the vitalistic philosophy of the traditional homeopathic community.

Throughout its 180-year history, homeopathy has been treated with indifference, contempt, and hostility. Its practitioners have consistently refused to be assimilated into the allopathic tradition, though they have been trained in the accepted approach to medicine before devoting themselves to homeopathic practice. As late as 1890 in the United States there were about 14,000 homeopaths in the country, as compared with 85,000 conventional physicians. At that time—and even now, when the number of homeopaths in the United States has declined to probably no more than 3,000—the homeopathic approach has always attracted more patients than the small number of practitioners would indicate. The outright battle between the regular physicians and homeopaths (almost every one of whom is a convert from conventional medicine) has raged for almost a hundred years, despite the refusal of the medical establishment to conduct a controlled and supervised investigation of homeotherapeutics. This despite the fact that as long ago as the European cholera epidemic of 1832, and in the ensuing epidemics of scarlet fever, dysentery, meningitis, and yellow fever, observers at the time testified that patients treated by homeopaths had a far higher recovery rate than those treated by the regular physicians, and that over the years many homeopathic remedies were adopted by orthodox physicians. Probably the most dramatic example of the latter is the use of nitroglycerine for certain cardiovascular diseases. Constantine Hering published his paper on the use of nitroglycerine in 1857; then twenty-five years later it appeared in the allopathic literature, after which it became one of the standard medications of the allopaths, who continue to use it widely today.

The current disaffection with conventional medicine, however, and especially the heightened consciousness of laymen who are displeased with and skeptical of the efficacy of brief, hurried visits to conventional physicians, followed so often by the prescription of "broad-spectrum" synthetic drugs, so many of which are likely to cause adverse reactions, makes homeopathy increasingly attractive. Indeed, the field is growing at this point, with an expansion of postgraduate education in homeopathy and parallel increases in the several professional homeopathic associations. In a day of sensitivity to holistic, humanistic principles, the fact that homeopathy's methods cannot directly harm patients, and that its practice has survived virtually intact for 180 years—implying the results its practitioners claimed—suggests that it may be possible now to build a bridge between conventional medicine and homeopathy that leads to a comprehensive integration of the strengths of both. For their part, homeopaths, while confident that their doctrines and techniques have, by virtue of enduring effectiveness and patient safety, truly proved the scientific basis for their practice through concrete and repeated performance, still do not claim to have all the answers. But their belief in their carefully elaborated system remains unshaken, and its possible integration with conventional medicine seems almost an imperative at this point in the history of health and medicine. Once again we appear to be at a juncture like that encountered in France in the late nineteenth century when the French statesman François Guizot was asked to ban homeopathy. He replied: "If homeopathy is a chimera or a valueless method, it will collapse. If, on the contrary, it represents an advance, it will spread whatever we do to stop it; and the Academy should desire this above all—as her mission is to stimulate scientific advances and encourage discoveries."

ROMEO: Your plantain leaf is excellent for that.
BENVOLIO: For what, I pray thee?
ROMEO: For your broken shin.

Shakespeare
Romeo and Juliet
Act 1, Scene 2

5.
MOTHER EARTH
MEDICINE:
The Almost Endless
Cycle of Usefulness

My friend Bill Webb has built a round house on a piece of high land that is part of a rattlesnake sanctuary overlooking Pfeiffer-Big Sur State Park a few miles north of Big Sur, California. It took him several years to complete the house, and as a base for operations he first built a cozy one-room cabin just below his house site, complete with a solar-cell-heated hot tub a few yards from the cabin.

That he would choose to live on a rattlesnake sanctuary, design and build a round house, and use solar power for even his temporary living quarters—all are typical of Bill's style: He is a self-reliant and self-confident Westerner, with an easy and matter-of-fact connection with natural things like sun, wood, land, and water. From the moment he picked out his house site, he planned that the land surrounding his eventual home would be a full-fledged herbarium, on which he would grow only those plants and flowers that could form a part of his life on the mountain: herbs that one could eat or use medicinally. His experienced eye had observed on his first visit that a vast assortment of such herbs were indigenous to the place, and he simply vowed that when all the construction was done, he would tend the entire hillside in such a way as to make it exclusively helpful to the natural life he planned to pursue on his land.

One day, as he was working on his property, it occurred to him that he had a guest coming for dinner for whom he would like to prepare a truly special dish. When he had first invited her, his plan had been to prepare an aromatic sauce served on fresh vermicelli. For some years he had developed a tasty recipe for his sauce, experimenting with this or that herb or seasoning until he reached a formula that pleased him. On the day in question he decided on still another experiment. One particular plant native to his land—an artemisia—had always delighted him with its aroma, and he reasoned that it might make a particularly redolent addition to his spaghetti sauce. When he went back to the cabin to begin cooking the meal, he plucked a few of the silvery green leaves from a plant, and when he got to the point of preparing his sauce, he threw them into the steaming pot of other ingredients. As the artemisia mixed with the sage, black pepper, tomatoes, and other herbs already slowly cooking, his nose told him that he had indeed made a rich discovery. The fumes coming off the steaming sauce were more appetizing than ever—pungent, sweet, and pervasive.

When his guest arrived, she commented on the rich and aromatic smells that suffused the cabin, so it was with special anticipation that Bill spooned the sauce over the pasta. He and his guest dug right in, and at first taste the experiment seemed a culinary triumph. But no more than four or five forkfuls later, each looked at the other with wonderment and shock. "I swear I felt my taste buds deaden," Bill said, "and almost immediately I felt my whole mouth go numb, as if I had been given several shots of Novocain by the dentist. My guest told me the same thing was happening to her, and I urged her to stop eating. I assured her nothing terrible or poisonous was going to happen to us, that we should just relax and sip a little wine until the anesthetic feeling passed. At the same time I had no idea how long this might take, but I assumed that the artemisia had caused the sensation, and had so pervaded the sauce that we couldn't avoid it and should stop eating. I was sure that the small quantity of leaves I had put in the sauce could not create a very long-lasting effect, so I quickly emptied our plates and served the salad. In about five or ten minutes we both felt our mouths returning to normal. The deadened effect passed and while eating a salad which I had dressed with vinegar and oil, I felt my taste come back. Within a half hour everything was all right, though I must say, the shock and disappointment put a real damper on the evening. She left early."

The next day Bill was again working on his new house, when he was approached by a neighbor complaining mightily about an attack of poison oak, the western version of the contact dermatitis caused elsewhere by poison ivy or poison sumac. The familiar weeping blisters that appear in clusters on the skin that has touched the ivy, oak, or sumac plant are always characterized by extreme itching, and though the popular belief that scratching the irritated area will spread the infection is incorrect (the "water" in the small blisters will not cause additional outbreaks; the blisters will appear only where oils from the plant have been in contact with the skin), the need to scratch is nerve-racking, and Bill's neighbor was in the throes of that feeling. Remembering his somewhat embarrassing dinner from the night before, Bill plucked a few leaves of artemisia and invited the woman into the cabin, saying that he might be able to relieve some of the itching. He boiled some water, and into it he dropped several clumps of artemisia leaves which he allowed to steep in the boiling water for ten minutes. When the mixture (which had some of the alluring aroma that had inspired Bill's fiasco of the previous night) had cooled to the point of skin comfort, Bill soaked some sterile gauze and gently laid the dressing on his neighbor's lower ribs, where the outbreak was most severe. Within a few moments she was bubbling with gratitude as the anesthetic lotion cooled her skin. Bill explained what he had done, and suggested that if the itching recurred she could prepare additional lotion herself and apply it as often as she wished. "My affection for the artemisia wasn't total folly," Bill thought, somewhat appeased. What he had chosen for food turned out to be useful as medicine.

The next day Bill's neighbor appeared again, this time happily agitated. "Look!" she cried, pointing to the place where Bill had applied dressings. The whole area of skin that had been pinkish red with irritation was distinctly paler, and even the blisters of her poison oak seemed smaller. She reported that she had applied the lotion only twice more since she had left Webb's cabin twenty-four hours before. Bill was as amazed as his "patient" and his pleasure was even greater two days later when the woman showed up again to display a complete cure of her attack.

When I heard this story, I was excited at Bill's discovery and determined to make the artemisia a part of my own pharmacopoeia. I got my chance less than two months later. My wife and I had returned to northwestern Connecticut from our trip to California, and in June, while gardening, Ann had come into the house with her arms covered with insect bites. We couldn't be sure which insects had been the culprits, but the itching sensation was profound and I saw an opportunity to repeat Bill's therapeutic success. We, too, have an artemisia plant on our property. We always called it "silver mound," but its botanical name is *Artemisia schmidtiana,* and it grows readily each year in attractive round clumps where we planted it next to the edge of the rock garden. I picked a few of the clumps, dropped them into boiling water and, when the mixture had cooled, repeated Bill's treatment with gauze pads. Alas, the results were far from dramatic. Ann reported that the lotion was pleasing but made no difference whatever in the itching, and after repeated treatments, it was clear that the magic of California artemisia was not to be found again in the Berkshire Hills of Connecticut.

My attempt to improvise on Bill's discovery illustrates the typical mixture of uncertainty, innocence, and hopefulness that surrounds our increased interest in herbal medicine. The whole notion of using common plants as medication has crept back into our world of options as part of the deepening skepticism we feel about synthetic drugs, invasive surgery, and overtechnological diagnostic procedures as part of our still inchoate attempt to reclaim responsibility for our own health or reduce our dependence on the scientific medicine that so often disappoints us. Yet, for the most part, we have no single identifiable, credible place to turn if we seek to use curative herbs. Traditional Chinese and Ayurvedic physicians use herbal medicines regularly; homeopaths dispense many medications which are derived from herbs; Native American healers customarily depend on herbal preparations as part of their standard treatment; there are ever increasing numbers of "naturopaths," whose medical practice is identified by their refusal to use *any* but natural substances—including herbs—in their treatment of illness and disease. And in much of the world, where traditional or ethnic medicine is still the dominant health care system, local herbs are the bedrock of treatment.

But all these lie outside the domain of scientific medicine, though the modern American physician, for example, might be surprised to discover that almost one fourth of the drugs he prescribes contain constituents derived directly from green plants. Those physicians have had little or no experience in the direct use of those plants and find it hard to believe that an infusion of chamomile tea can lull a restless patient to sleep just as effectively as a little white pill. The pharmaceutical companies, of course, do little to dispel the atmosphere of skepticism and disbelief that surrounds physicians throughout their training and practice. The research budgets of those companies, which probably total $1 billion dollars annually, include no more than $200,000 for plant research. This may result from profit considerations to a great extent, but it also reflects the fact that the "mind" of the pharmaceutical industry reflects the narrow construction of modern medicine that considers the cause of disease to be internal chemical distortion, and that cure can be achieved only by devising a chemical drug that will supress or inactivate the chemical process that is thought to cause the patient's malady.

The mood of the modern patient who finds this formulation limited may be resistant and self-reliant, but the alternatives, when it comes to herbal medicines, are not clear-cut. We are at the point in human history where self-education and experimentation are part of our assumption of responsibility. We can hope that more physicians will become receptive to the reconsideration and rediscovery of the healing power of green plants, just as they appear to be welcoming more information and training in the significance of nutrition in the treatment of illness and disease. But before this can become standard and universal, we must recapture much of the neglected sixty-thousand-year history of the use of herbs in medical practice.

The reason for my failure to duplicate Bill Webb's healing with artemisia became obvious as I pursued my studies. Of the almost 180 species that have at one time or another been classified, there are at least nine distinct species of artemisia growing in the United States, the most common being *Artemisia absinthium* (wormwood), *Artemisia frigida* (a source of camphor), *Artemisia schmidtiana* (silver mound), *Artemisia abrotanum* (southernwood), *Artemisia vulgaris* (mugwort). It soon became clear that despite Bill's success with its western cousin, the feathery silver foliage of our northeastern artemisia will remain primarily a decorative border plant.

The best known artemisia is the *Artemisia absinthium,* or wormwood, which is mentioned in the Bible (it was used by the Jews as one of the bitter herbs eaten during the Passover) and was described as well in one of the oldest written herbals, the Ebers Papyrus of about 1500 B.C. That manuscript names more than 125 plants, with hundreds of prescriptions for disease and accident cures or alleviation that sound remarkably similar to modern complaints: burns, constipation, catarrh, cystitis, tumors, eye and throat infections, and so on. At possibly an even earlier time, the Chinese recorded a materia medica, the *Shen Nung Ben Tsao,* which listed more than 300 medicines and described their therapeutic properties.

Under the Tang Dynasty (7th century A.D.) more than two thousand scholars were enlisted in the revision of the ancient materia medica, and a revised edition was published in 659 A.D. About nine hundred years later, in 1578, China's greatest naturalist, Li Shih-chen published his own magnum opus, called *Ben Tsao Kung Mu* (The Chinese Pharmacopoeia). Li had devoted twenty-seven years of his seventy-five-year life to his work, traveling over most of China, interviewing peasants as well as scientists, and ultimately he collected 1,892 different kinds of medical materials, of which were 1,094 were botanical species. (His book also contained more than 1,000 standard medical prescriptions, many of which are still used at the present time.)

There is evidence that all over the world four thousand years ago the usefulness of plants as medicine was not only being discovered, but also the detailed knowledge of such plants was being organized and passed on from generation to generation. The roots, bark, and seeds of plants were being used everywhere, and it is one of the provocative mysteries of such experimentation that when modes of travel finally developed and the peoples of the earth finally began to visit each other, the claims made regarding the particular healing properties of certain herbs from one region were identical with those claimed for the same herbs in another area.

Just why early humans assumed plants to be curative is not known. Speculation ranges from the notion that man simply imitated the animals of his time to the idea that human beings possess what René Dubos calls a "medical instinct," a mechanism of consciousness that apparently leads us to assume that nature has provided for our needs and that only deduction from trial and error is needed to create the universal materia medica.

Like Jung's discovery that all people, even those whom history insists could not have interacted, visualize the same archetypal symbols and make them part of their psychological, artistic, and cultural life, the belief that nature has provided plants as medicines is ubiquitous. In addition to the elaborate Egyptian papyrus and the Chinese catalogue of herbal remedies, the Ayurvedic medicine of India, for example, has developed a pharmacopoeia of some two thousand plants, and these herbal remedies still provide the most widely used treatment for the peoples of the Indian subcontinent.

The Hebrews, Arabs, Babylonians, Greeks, Romans, and Persians all recorded the balms and remedies that derived from their native plant life, and currently familiar herbs like ginseng, licorice, cumin, peppermint, and fennel appear throughout the ancient writings as specifics for certain accidents and illnesses.

The modern attitude toward plant drugs is largely colored by an indulgent amusement at our "primitive" ancestors, a condescension to the ingenuity of their fumbling experiments and childlike discoveries. We forget that nature's healing plants are at the heart of the catalogue of healing substances we use. Only in the past forty years, for instance, has the anciently trusted quinine been replaced as a cure for malaria, and to this day our technological ingenuity has failed to improve on the painkilling properties of morphine, one of the active principles of the poppy known as *Papaver somniferum;* rauwolfia (snakeroot), a basic substance in Indian medical literature, introduced to the Western world the much abused concept of tranquilizers; iodine derived from seaweed; curare, still a valuable handmaiden of modern anesthesia; and penicillin itself, one of the most common substances in the modern pharmacopoeia—all these came to us from the ancient traditions of using plants that grow near to us in nature. The relative of the wormwood that Bill Webb discovered to be so helpful in treating poison oak was a drug recommended by Moses Maimonides in the thirteenth century as a diuretic (a stimulator of the secretion of urine) and is still prescribed for that purpose.

In the New World the early colonists brought with them a body of knowledge about herbs that heal, only to discover that the natives of both American continents already had developed a quite sophisticated herbal medicine, including narcotics and analgesics. The first herbal in the Americas, the Badianus Manuscript, sometimes called the "Aztec Herbal," was written in the sixteenth century in the Nahuatl language of the Indians of Mexico, later translated into both Latin and Spanish, and represented the accumulated materia medica of hundreds of years of common usage; and once again the universality of healing herbs was confirmed. Wormwood, cayenne pepper, hyssop (which is mentioned in the Gospel of St. John [19:29]: "Now there was set a vessel full of vinegar: and they filled a sponge with vinegar, and put it upon hyssop, and put it to his mouth"), and the various plantains all appear in the Aztec Herbal, where they are recognized as therapeutic for many of the same conditions that are described in older texts from far distant corners of the earth.

By the middle of the nineteenth century, at least in the United States and Europe, almost 80 percent of the medicines used were derived from plants; today almost half the curatives in the average family's medicine chest are manufactured from either organic or inorganic chemicals, and only 30 percent are plant-based. Ours has been the century that launched the chemical era; we have turned our skills to the synthesis of the active principles that have been isolated from herbs, and not until the discovery of penicillin (produced from, among other sources, a mold that grows on the same hyssop leaves that figured in Holy Scripture and the Aztec Herbal) was any brake at all put on the headlong commitment to synthetic products. If there is now anything that can be called the "herbal revolution" it is a renaissance, encouraged by a new awareness that the individual must reclaim some of the responsibility for his own health from the scientific experts of modern medicine, and an understanding that although the benefits of man-made drugs are indisputable, the manufacturers of synthetic substances have not produced cures for such pervasive modern afflictions as asthma, heart trouble, arthritis, insanity, and cancer. Furthermore, the clinical era has also introduced the concept of "side effects," which in their most extreme form have become the hallmark of iatrogenic, or physician-induced illnesses and disabilities. Ranging from minor but irritating allergic responses to aspirin, penicillin, and cortisone to the tragedy and scandal of the deformed babies born to mothers who had taken the drug thalidomide to quell the nausea of pregnancy, the spectrum of possible negative reactions to synthetic medicines has become common knowledge. The fear of such apparently unpredictable effects from drug use has combined with the current mood of self-reliance, ecological consciousness, and increasing sophistication about nutrition to magnify the interest in traditional herbal medicine as the "people's pharmacy," echoing Thoreau's aphorism that "man may esteem himself happy when that which is his food is also his medicine."

The new back-to-nature movement in the United States has passed the point of being merely chic. The sale of health food products totaled $144 billion in 1979, representing a 40 percent jump over the year before. The sale of herb-related products accounted for 10.4 percent of that total, second only to health vitamin products. The herbal tea industry alone had sales of $120 million in 1979, almost double its volume in 1978. (This is still only about one sixth of the $750 million black leaf tea business, but the growth of the latter industry has for some years been limited to less than 10 percent in any one year and many of the national brand name tea makers introduced their own herbal tea assortments in 1980 and are spending staggering amounts on their advertising to this day.)

The dramatic growth in the popularity of herbal teas is clearly related to the increasing medical evidence of caffeine's harmful effects. Caffeine is a basic ingredient of black leaf tea that is absent in almost all herbal teas. Americans have been consuming 35 million pounds of caffeine per year for some years. There are almost 100 milligrams of the substance in an average cup of coffee, and about 50 milligrams in a typical serving of cola drink or tea. Caffeine has several effects: It is a diuretic; it is a "central nervous system stimulant," providing in that role a wide variety of effects from mild irritability to severe insomnia; and in studies during the late 1970s caffeine was more spectacularly implicated as a possible cause of birth defects and cystic breast disease in women.

There is one plant, *Camellia thea,* that is, strictly speaking, the tea plant. But the word "tea" has slipped generally into a larger meaning to describe any brew made by mixing any solid substance with boiling or very hot water. This process is called an *infusion,* and this is the most often used method of preparing any herb for medicinal use. In preparing a medical infusion, the common practice is to pour two cups of boiling water onto one ounce of the dried herb (the equivalent of one tablespoonful) or over one loose handful of the fresh herbs. Herbalists are careful to use only enamel, glass, or ceramic containers for this process, since metal pots, particularly aluminum, interact chemically with herbs, creating impure mixtures. An infusion is allowed to steep for at least ten minutes to assure that the active ingredients of the plant—vitamins and other volatile components—have been extracted. The infusion is poured after ten minutes, and honey may be added to taste. This mixture is the so-called "standard brew" in herbal medicine, and a small cupful three or four times a day is the usual prescription.

The tradition of soothing teas is part of the grandmother lore of every culture. Belief in the healing power of an infusion is as old as water itself, and the nursing instinct to prepare hot tea for the ailing patient extends from Peter Rabbit's mother, who when "Peter was not very well during the evening . . . put him to bed and made some camomile tea: One tablespoonful to be taken at bedtime," to the wife of the redoubtable detective, Inspector Maigret, who sniffles through the stories of Georges Simenon, often taking to his bed with heavy cold symptoms. In *Maigret's Dead Man,* for instance, he uses his affliction to retreat from his office and stay at home where "his wife would baby him. She would walk around on tiptoe . . . his colleagues came to visit him or telephone. Everybody was patient with him. They inquired after his health, and in exchange for a certain number of herb teas, which he drank with a grimace, he got his solicitous wife to give him a few hot toddies." (This latter, of course is still another form of infusion.)

Another method of preparing herbs is a *decoction,* used when the material to be extracted is a bitter or mineral salt. In this case the herb— the entire herb, the seed, or root or bark—is soaked in *cold* water for several hours and then brought to a boil and simmered for a half hour. In a decoction, the proportion is one ounce of dried plant material to two cups of water, and because the decoction is stronger than an infusion, the appropriate dose is one-half cup before meals. However, a decoction is usually taken cool rather than hot, and again, to avoid the grimaces of Maigret, honey may be used as a sweetener.

Without honey both infusions and decoctions may be used externally, just as Bill Webb and I did with our respective artemisias. Technically, the applications we used were *fomentations,* because we used the infusion full-strength, dipped a cloth in the tea, and wrung out the excess moisture. This is the most useful way to use either an infusion or a decoction in treating skin irritations, headaches, or insect bites.

A variation on the decoction is called an *embrocation,* the result of diluting a decoction in a gallon of water, used on those occasions where a large quantity is required for such injuries as a sprained ankle, foot, wrist, or finger. Embrocations are always used hot, and unsweetened.

Still another method of preparing curative herbs is the *tincture.* One part of pure alcohol or brandy is added to two ounces of dried plant material (or a large handful of fresh herbs) in a glass jar. The jar is capped tightly—the rubber-gasketed Mason jar is useful in this case—and turned upside down. Once or twice a day for a week, the jar is shaken vigorously, after which the mixture is strained and the liquid replaced in the jar where it will keep its strength for up to six months. The recommended dose for a tincture is only one tablespoonful to a wineglass of water, once or twice a day. The tincture method is used in conventional pharmacology, too, in preparing alcoholic or hydroalcoholic (water and alcohol combined) solutions of medicinal substances such as iodine, although usually these mixtures are obtained by using a suitable solvent along with the alcohol or water to achieve the appropriate dilution.

In addition to the storage jar in which herbs can be safely kept for long periods, honey may be used to preserve herbs or herbal mixtures. The preservative qualities of honey have been known for centuries, perhaps the most dramatic proof being the discovery of a quantity of Asian honey which lay underground in Egypt for about twenty-five hundred years, and which when tested was found to be remarkably close to normal, fresh honey in color, consistency, and stickiness. In herbal medicine, honey is used either as a direct preservative, by placing dried herbal materials into a quantity of honey for storage, where it will hold the freshness of the herbs for a month or two, or, more commonly, to make a cough syrup. This method is called a *standard brew concentrate,* and is prepared by first making a concentrated infusion (tea), consisting of eight ounces of the herb to twelve ounces of water. After infusing this mixture for fifteen or twenty minutes, it is strained, and an equal amount of honey is added and stirred. The herbs most commonly used to prepare such a syrup are horehound and coltsfoot, either together or individually, and the recommended dose is two teaspoons in one-half glass of warm water, taken three or four times a day.

The standard brew concentrate—eight ounces of herb infused with twelve ounces of water—can also be used to prepare a pleasant flavoring to add to such bitter-tasting herbs as wormwood and boneset. Juniper berries are a favorite ingredient for such a flavoring agent, but wine (which also preserves herbal medicines for several months) may be used.

For external use, herbs are usually prepared as a *poultice*—the "mustard plaster," applied to the chest for coughs and colds, being the classical example. Fresh or dried herbs are chopped fine and moistened with apple cider vinegar and then mixed with whole wheat flour or cooked barley as a binder for the mixture, the formula being one part of the herb mixture to three parts of the binder. The mixture is then spread on a moist cloth, the ends and sides of which are folded over. The skin to be treated is oiled lightly, and the poultice laid over it with either a piece of plastic or a heating pad (on a low setting) placed on top of the poultice to help retain the heat. The use of poultices is described in what has often been called the world's oldest medical text, a small Sumerian clay tablet that has been dated from the Third Dynasty of Ur, around 2158–2008 B.C., or even earlier. Of the fifteen prescriptions listed on the tablet, twelve are for external use and eight of these are plasters or poultices. The "drugs" used with these bandages are not unfamiliar. One prescription, for example, reads, "pound together dried wine dregs, juniper and prunes; pour beer on the mixture. Then rub (the affected parts) with oil and bind on as a plaster." Almost as old as the poultice, and sometimes used as a dressing with a plaster, is the *salve,* or ointment. Whether the basic ingredient was ox grease, ibis grease, lion grease, or grease from the foot of a hippopotamus, the various medical papyri dating from as far back as 1900 B.C. all make much of the use of grease and honey salves for the dressing of wounds. The well-known passages in the Book of Jeremiah (8:21–22; 46:11) are only a part of the evidence suggesting that myrrh and other resins were among the most common drugs used:

> I am wounded at the sight of my people's wounds,
> I go like a mourner, overcome with horror.
> Is there no balm in Gilead, no physician there? . . ."
>
> Go up into Gilead and fetch balm,
> O virgin people of Egypt.
> You have tried many remedies, all in vain;
> No skin shall grow over your wounds.

Even though the biblical text has usually been interpreted metaphorically, the reality, borne out by the records of ancient Mesopotamia, Egypt, and Greece, was that balms and salves were the stuff of early surgical medicine. Looking back with the analytical eye of modern science, we might think that our ancestors knew, either intuitively or consciously, that what mends and heals gashes in plants and trees might also heal wounds in people. Perhaps they were driven to mitigate the fetid odor of wounds and used the balm of a fragrant frankincense sap oozing from a wounded tree, or they may have observed that resins are among the few products of nature that never decay and hoped to transmit this quality to the wounds of human skin. It is not likely that in any but an unconscious way the ancients could have known an even better reason for the uses of resins like myrrh: many act as a bacteriostatic agent against such typical microorganisms as *Staphylococcus aureus.* Even plants that are not resinous earn their way into ancient pharmacopoeias, presumably on the basis of their fragrance; thyme, favored in the Hippocratic text, still has a place in modern pharmacology, the essence of thyme (crystalline thymol) being used in laboratory solutions to preserve them from bacteria and mildew.

In any case, salves prepared from herbs remain a basic and useful method to treat abrasions, minor burns, insect bites and stings, and contact dermatitis, the increasingly common skin irritation resulting from living in a world of irritants, synthetic chemicals, and pollutants. To prepare a salve, fresh or dried herbs are covered with water, brought to a boil, and simmered for thirty minutes. The liquid is then strained, and to it is added an equal amount of olive or safflower oil. Again, the mixture is simmered, this time until the water has evaporated in steam and only the oil is left. To this is added enough beeswax to give the mixture the consistency of a salve, and while hot the mixture is poured into glass or plastic jars (with tight covers), in which the salves will last up to a year or more.

A vocabulary developed over the centuries to describe the particular or compound properties the salves had been found to possess. The most common qualities are colloquially familiar: "Aromatic," "astringent," for example, are words used in general as well as medical conversation. But there are over forty summary terms used by herbalists and naturopathic physicians to designate the special properties that commend herbs to specific uses. Some of the most relevant terms are:

Alterative:	Nonspecific but persistent action which improves the general functioning of body parts and, when taken over a long period of time, favorably alters the course of an ailment.
Anodyne:	Allays pain.
Anthelmintic:	Eliminates or destroys intestinal worms.
Antiperiodic:	Prevents cyclical return of a disease.
Antiseptic:	Destroys and/or checks growth of harmful bacteria.
Antispasmodic:	Relieves or stops spasms, convulsions, and cramps.
Aperient:	Acts as a gentle, nonpurging laxative.
Astringent:	Has a drawing or contracting effect on soft tissue.
Carminative:	Expels gas from the alimentary canal.
Chologogue:	Increases the flow of bile.
Demulcent:	Soothes and protects irritated tissue, particularly the mucous membranes of the body.
Deobstructant:	Opens the natural passages of the body.
Diaphoretic:	Produces involuntary perspiration.

Diuretic:	Increases secretion and flow of urine.
Emetic:	Induces vomiting.
Emmenagogue:	Promotes menstrual flow.
Emollient:	Softens and soothes inflamed tissue.
Expectorant:	Promotes discharge of mucus from respiratory tract.
Febrifuge:	Reduces and abates fever.
Hemostatic:	Stops bleeding.
Hepatic:	Affects the liver.
Laxative:	A mild purgative.
Mucilaginous:	Having a gelatinous or adhesive quality.
Nervine:	Acts to soothe the nerves.
Parturient:	Helps to induce childbirth.
Pectoral:	Clears and relieves respiratory tract.
Purgative:	Causes thorough emptying of the bowels.
Refrigerant:	Reduces body heat.
Rubefacient:	Increases circulation and produces slight reddening of the skin.
Sedative:	Relieves tension, soothes the nerves.
Stimulant:	Produces temporary quickening of a vital process.
Stomachic:	Promotes gastric digestion.
Styptic:	Arrests bleeding.
Tonic:	Invigorates and strengthens the entire body.
Vermifuge:	Expels worms.
Vulnerary:	Heals wounds.

(These terms are used in Part II of this book, where selected herbs and their specific uses are described.)

Since these definitions evolved as a kind of shorthand to facilitate the research and writing of professionals, their technical nature is rarely a problem for a layman. Not so the names of herbs themselves and their botanical classification. As every gardener knows, the labeling of trees, flowers, and plants engenders the same sort of confusion and false expectations that occurred to me when I tried to replicate Bill Webb's medical use of artemisia.

In a sense, all plants can be said to have a scientific name, a common name, and, in most cases, several nicknames, the latter being usually the physically descriptive local name applied by people in different parts of the world as they discovered new plants in their area. By the seventeenth and eighteenth centuries, when the study of plants intensified all over the world, the difficulties in relying on common names became a troublesome obstacle to scholarship. When botanists throughout Europe, parts of Asia, and America began to exchange information through written journals and letters, the absence of a universal plant nomenclature made it difficult to establish the identity of the plants being discussed. Gradually, Latin, known by most scholars, became accepted for naming plants, and animals as well. The Latin names already given by Romans were adopted, and new plants were assigned new Latin names.

The major figure in this development was the Swedish botanist Linnaeus, who changed his own surname, Linné, to the Latinized version by which he is known. His recognition, for example, that there are many kinds of roses led him to the idea that merely adding adjectives to *rosa* would become unwieldy and awkward, so he hit on the idea of giving each rose a second name, often descriptive, which could be used exclusively for that rose. Thus, a specific white rose became *Rosa alba,* and while there may be other white roses, each would have its own exclusive name as well. This system gave rise to the convention, when cataloguing or describing herbs, to use not only the general name of the herb, but also its common variations or nicknames, its Latin name, the family of plants to which the species belongs, and an initial or abbreviation to indicate the botanist who first described the species. Thus, the common herb called St.-John's-wort is the plant *hypericum perforatum* L. ("L." being the initial of Linnaeus), belonging to the family called Guttiferae, and known variously as God's wonderplant, devil's scourge, llamath weed, goat weed, grace of god, hundred holes, herb John, rosin rose, terrestrial sun, and amber touch-and-heal.

In this case, the common name probably dates from the Middle Ages when favorite plants or flowers were often consecrated to or named after a saint, especially if the plant was believed to possess medicinal properties. The choice of the saint was usually determined by the month in which the flower bloomed, and it seems likely that it was monks, who spent much of their time in gardening and who were the chief herbalists of their time, who named many of the plants to honor religious heroes. St.-John's-wort usually blossoms near the summer solstice, and since the birthday of St. John is thought to be the twenty-fourth of June, many people still believe that if sprays of the plant are hung in the window on that date they will keep away "ghosts, devils, and thunderbolts." Furthermore, the oil glands of the plant, which can be seen if the leaf is held up to the light, secrete a red fluid which is called "St. John's blood" and is believed by some to spot the leaves on August 29th, the date that John the Baptist was beheaded.

The subtle details of plants like St.-John's-wort that have been so central to their naming reflect the observation of, and experimentation with, plants that have been carried out for centuries all over the world. Every plant has several parts that may be used in preparing botanical medicines, and only the close attention to the effects of using various components of the plant could have created the traditional prescriptions that have endured for so many years. The essential parts of all plants are their roots, stems, leaves, and flowers. The "whole herb," or all of it that grows above ground, is the useful part of some plants; the root, or that part which grows underground, is the valuable part of others. The formation and characteristics of these parts are the details by which they are identified and classified.

There are, for example, four common root forms with distinctive shapes: The taproot (usually straight and narrow like a carrot), the napiform root (shaped like a turnip), the fusiform root (spindle-shaped), and the familiar tuberous root, with several rounded swellings. Some herbs have exclusively underground stems, known as rhizomes. (See illustrations.)

The stems and branches of plants are essentially of two kinds. Those with stems and branches that rise above the ground are known as "caulescent," (having a "true" stem), and this describes most herbs that grow in the temperate climates. The other kind of stem formation—the "acaulescent" or "stemless"—is typified by the common crocus or the violet plant. The underground rhizome root also develops spreading underground stems which put down roots at intervals from the original plant and send up leaves and flowers along this path. The various clovers are typical of the rhizome spread.

The arrangement of the caulescent stems and branches is a useful clue to identifying the plant. For the most part, herbs have "true," erect stems, but there are four variations of that formation: Diffuse stems spread loosely over the ground in all directions; declined stems bend to one side; decumbent stems lie flat on the ground as though they cannot support the weight of the plant; prostrate or recumbent stems are strong but also lie along the ground; creeping or repent stems lie on the ground, but put down new roots as they grow horizontally.

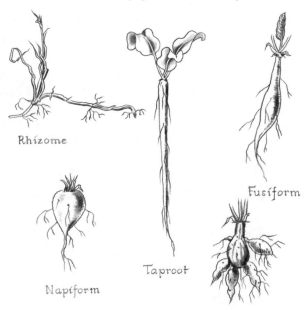

Rhizome

Fusiform

Napiform

Taproot

Tuberous

The "herbal revolution," as noted, has made dried herb products much more generally available. But for those who either are curious as to what parts of the plants are used in the dried products or would like to gather or grow their own herbs, it is worth noting that in herbal medicine three parts of the plant are usually used: the root and the underground stem (rhizome); what is usually called the "whole herb," meaning the stem, leaf, and flower; and, finally, the bark. Roots are best collected in the early spring, before the aboveground parts have begun to appear, or in late autumn when the foliage has died down. The "whole herb" should be gathered in the summer, when the plant is beginning to bloom and the important essence of the plant is in its foliage and blossom. The bark is collected in the spring when the sap is moving up from the roots to nourish the leaves.

The gathering up of the fruits of the earth is part of the recorded history of all peoples and is usually thought of as an aspect of religious gratitude to whatever supernatural deity has provided food and medicine for human use. The general rules that now govern herb gathering are based on understanding the periods in which the respective parts of plants are at their peak. Traditionally, those who collect herbal materials have been even more specific and formal, and what appeared to be religious habit has now been discovered to be precise knowledge. For instance, the yield of morphine from the poppy at 9 A.M. is often four times the yield obtained twelve hours later, and the same diurnal variation has been shown with various other plants, including deadly nightshade (belladonna), henbane, stramonium (thorn apple), and mandrake. Likewise, variations in the exact stage of germination cause wide differences in the active principle of the plant. In the case of the periwinkle, for example, a plant that has been used in a great many countries in the treatment of diabetes (and which is being seriously investigated for its possible effectiveness in treating leukemia), there are virtually no active principles in the seeds. But they do appear during germination and within three weeks are present throughout the plant—only to disappear, and then reappear around eight weeks later. The old-time herbalists, in other words, knew what they were doing when they specified detailed schedules for the collection of healing plants. (Not only timing, but the attitude of the herb gatherer has also figured in the tradition. The American Indian medicine man gathers his herbs quite ceremoniously, praying over the plants before picking them, taking only what he needs and being careful to make his words and movements gentle and respectful.)

Many herbs can be grown easily in the various temperature zones in the United States, and methods for cultivating, drying, and storing the herbs are covered in several of the books described in the bibliography in the back of this book. (Nelson Coon's *Using Plants for Healing* and Adele G. Dawson's *Health, Happiness, and the Pursuit of Herbs* are particularly useful in this regard.) But most of us will want to purchase medicines that

have been processed commercially, since different parts of the plant ma-
ture at different seasons, and collecting the medicinal part at the right
time requires special attention.

The processing of medical plants is directed not only at making them
more readily available but also toward increasing the efficacy of the plant.
Cleaning the plant, for example, has been found to facilitate storage, and
proper cleaning methods also reduce or eliminate toxicity. In general, the
processing of herbs consists of sorting, washing, slicing, and drying the
medicinal plants, after which they are stored in sealed glass jars or
wooden cases, from which they are dispensed in small, individual quantities. Herbs, of course, lose strength with age, and should be discarded
after twelve to fifteen months. (Throwing herbs away need not be as
wasteful as it sounds. In the summer, "leftover" herbs may be sprinkled
around garden plants, dug into the soil, or added to the compost pile.
Many herbs—wormwood, southernwood, mugwort, tansy, rue, and hyssop, for instance—have specific value in the garden as insect repellents.)

The almost endless cycle of usefulness of plants makes it all the more
remarkable that herbal remedies are still considered by so many to be
"primitive" or "unscientific." The sequence by which plants are used as
food by one of *our* basic foods—animals—and themselves are equally
central to our own diet as vegetables, does not suggest to us that when we
use plants medicinally we are employing active organic substances which
are in harmony with our own physical composition. Our love affair with
industrial chemistry, which is based on the belief that pharmaceutical
processes extract what chemists believe to be the "active ingredient" of
plants and then mix it with synthetic materials in the laboratory, has led
us to fill our medicine chests with drugs that are invariably accompanied
by warnings that these products "may cause dizziness, blurring of vision,
diarrhea, depression, decrease of mental activity, decreased libido, urti-
caria, and eczema," while all around us grow plants that we may use with
their chemical constituents intact, at far less risk of unwanted rashes,
increased heartbeats, breathing difficulties, or drowsiness. This is not to
say that plants are uniformly pure and without threats of toxicity, but by
and large, the chemical risks in botanical medicine are minimal if common
sense and widely published cautions are heeded. (See "Notes on Using
Herbs" in Part II of this book.)

But unlike the "father of medicine," Hippocrates, who urged that we
"look to the country and the season before deciding on treatment," we
have come to distrust or dismiss the immediate environment as a source
of healing in favor of packaged and overprocessed substances that are to
medicines what packaged and overprocessed foods have become to the
simple, natural fruits of our gardens. As with food, the principle of "con-
venience" has replaced efficacy as the standard for selecting drugs. This is
especially shocking when you consider that in one recent year alone in
Great Britain, the number of admissions to the hospital for treatment of

adverse reactions to synthetic drugs exceeded 100,000. This amazing figure should not be seized upon as yet another proof of the inadequacy of
the modern physician, for an equally astounding statistic—the existence
currently of over 30,000 separate synthetic pharmaceutical drugs—should
make it clear that it is quite impossible for any doctor to have sufficient
knowledge to assure the use of them without high risk. That we have
benefitted from over a century of almost exclusive emphasis on synthe-
sizing "miracle drugs" is unquestionable. But during that same time we
have been persistently reminded that nature has also built into us a capacity for counteracting their effects by inducing resistance to them, and
despite the gains of chemical progress we are still without drugs that cure
many of the diseases of modern civilization. Without abandoning the
developments in manufactured drugs, it now appears especially inviting
to redress the imbalance and give equal research attention and hope to the
botanical riches which surround us, and add them once more to the comprehensive pharmacopoeia that nature has provided for us. The plants
with which we share the same climate, seasons, air, soil, and water are the
source of the substances we need to maintain health, and the sixty thousand years in which they have been tested should be as reassuring to us as
the most sophisticated tests of the modern laboratory. For as it is written
in the Book of Revelations (22:2), "In the midst of the street of it, and on
either side of the river, was there the tree of life, which bore twelve
manner of fruits, and yielded her fruit every month; and the leaves of the
tree were for the healing of the nations."

I have learned never to underestimate
the capacity of the human mind and body to
regenerate—even when the prospects seem
most wretched. The life-force may be the
least understood force on earth.

Norman Cousins
Anatomy of an Illness

6.
FIELDS OF HEALTH:
The Forces-of-Energy Medicine

Ethertricity	Mana	Manna
Astral light	Élan vital	Eckankar
Entelechy	Spiritus	Baraka
Arealoha	Tondi	Psychotronic energy
Eloptic energy	Reiki	Tinh
Elima	Animal magnetism	Mungo
Dynamis	Vis naturalis	Kerei
El	Mumia	Orenda
Digin	Prana	Numen
Maxpe	Ch'i	Vital fluid
Hullo	Ki	Odic force
Wakan	Ka	Nervous ether
Huna	Pneuma	Cosmoelectricity
Archeus	Syntropy	Vis medicatrix naturae
Physis	Biocosmic energy	Paraelectricity
X-force	Bioplasma	

This list of forty-seven words contains only some of the terms that have been used across time and around the world to designate the fundamental life-force or energy that animates all living organisms. Human curiosity and imagination have always sought to give a name to what in most religions is accepted as the "spirit," the human share of the divine spark, the unseen quality that links humanity with its gods and provides the motive force for all creation. So long as the concept of an energetic essence in the universe was part of the act of religious faith, it could be credited or regretted for all the inexplicable events that befell human beings, including, of course, "miracle" recoveries from illness or premature deaths. In the face of such mysterious power one could only be humble or accepting.

As Vine Deloria puts it, "The observations and experiences of primitive peoples were so acute that they were able to recognize a basic phenomenon of the natural world religiously rather than scientifically. They felt power but did not measure it. Today we measure power but are unable to feel it except on extremely rare occasions. We conclude that energy forms the basic constituent of the universe through experimentation, and the existence of energy is truly a conclusion of scientific experimentation. For primitive peoples, on the other hand, the presence of energy and power is the starting point of their analysis and understanding of the natural world. It is their cornerstone for further exploration."

For most of the world, under the spell of science as a new religion, the idea of exploring what has been "merely" metaphysical has been left to those who persist in some religious faith in the life-force. Since that life-force does not submit to the laws of physics and chemistry that have dominated the modern view of the world and human nature, it has been relegated to the role of artifact, a kind of historical curio. In the practice of medicine, dealing with the idea of energy has been left to the "soft" branches of science: psychology and psychiatry. To many surgeons or internists or gastroenterologists, the aspect of energy sometimes called "vitality" is confined to the measurement of the comparably named "vital signs," such as heart rate, breathing pattern, or blood pressure. Any negative deviations from normal rates in these measurements that cannot be explained by physiology are considered "mental states," involving such imprecise and unscientific matters as attitudes, or hopes, or purposes, or even meaningfulness. Even the most rigid scientist of medicine will acknowledge that he has seen cases where his usually reliable physiological measurements cannot explain how a patient can be so remarkably functional, or in some cases, even alive. But the scientist's shrugging humility in the face of such an observation does not usually provoke his exploration. As Deloria implies, invisible and immeasurable phenomena are not on most agendas of science-bound medicine.

In the past fifty years a number of influences have come to challenge that traditional position. Clearly the most dramatic has been the evolution of Einsteinian and quantum physics, one of whose basic and confirmable findings has been that all matter is energy, all matter that appears static exists in a dynamic field, and that this activity of matter is indeed the very essence of its being. As Fritjof Capra says, "The existence of matter and its activity cannot be separated. They are but different aspects of the same space-time reality."

The emergence of this new physics has been taking place during the same period that has seen the rediscovery and reexamination of philosophical and medical systems that have *always* assumed the indivisibility of matter and energy: Taoist and Buddhist philosophy and the therapeutics based on them, Hindu religion and its related medical practices, and more recent vitalistic theories such as homeopathy. All these not only embrace the notion of the universal vital force manifesting in all living things, a vital force beyond the microscopes and meters of conventional science, but a force clearly evident nevertheless in the efforts of the human body to heal itself, to become whole. Albert Szent-Györgi (who twice won the Nobel Prize in biology) calls this immeasurable striving the "innate drive in living matter to perfect itself," and has shown in his own work with muscle protein and motor nerve cells that a kind of inherent "wisdom" can be confirmed in all living organisms and may explain the tendency of such organisms to strive for higher and higher levels of organization. This is a faint echo of Smuts's theory of holism, and though Szent-Györgi is less insistent about claiming this "drive" and "wisdom" as *the* universal force in natural evolution, he clearly has found many ways to express the principle even in the language of accredited science.

But by merely using the language of physical science, the advocates of a central life energy do not convince the skeptic. The history of energy theory is known to be bound up with myth and religion, the belief in a "spiritual" or "astral" plane in the human being. Modern, conventional science cannot accept the idea that by addressing curative treatment to that spectral aspect, we can hope for some transfer of the healing process to the physical plane. The Navajo who rises, healed, from the sand-painting and chanting ritual of his ancestors is not persuasive. The asthma patient who is relieved of his symptoms by ingesting homeopathic remedies in which no measurable portion of chemical material is present does not persuade the scientist. The person whose stomach spasms are relieved by fine acupuncture needles inserted in his legs does not answer the doubts. Commonly, the explanations of the physics- and chemistry-bound observer most often rely on crediting the placebo effect or the patients' "belief" in the efficacy of the cure. That this phenomenon *itself* is unexplainable—thus leaving open the question of what *really* effected the cure—does not open the question, but rather closes it with the finality of a Latin word (to give it the stature of science?) that puts the mysterious power into a labeled category.

As Richard Grossinger has pointed out in his remarkable book, *Planet Medicine*, " 'Energy medicine' is the name for an ostensible basic property of the universe, a property integrated in living systems, or in the living aspect of all systems, a property we have either lost in our millennia-long materialization of the cosmos, never known and thus seek in some future science, or have in our midst and resist and do not know how to define. We may not, in the end, choose to call it 'energy medicine,' but at this stage of things, 'energy medicine' calls into action the cluster of computing systems and advocacies we would want. . . ."

Whichever of these speculations may turn out to be true, there are a wide range of ancient and new therapeutic systems that are based on the assumption that the life energy, either as part of the mind-body complex or as a function of the "higher" or "astral" plane of existence, can be worked with, manipulated by hand or gesture or word, and that these systems can be taught to ordinary people for their own self-governance and self-healing.

Of these systems, several seem to me more appropriate than others for use as adjunctive therapies in conventional medical care. For example, zone therapy, or reflexology, which has roots in ancient systems that posited the idea that the whole body is represented in the hands and feet, has been refined and adapted in the past fifty years into a formal massage and manipulation system in which a considerable number of people have received extensive training. But it is difficult to extract a piece of this procedure and make it a complementary treatment in a clinical setting. As pleasurable as a comprehensive hand or foot massage may be, it does not fit handily into current medical practice. (A brief description of it and instructions are in Part II, but only as a guide to a pleasant form of self-care and caring interaction.)

Likewise, systems such as radionics, radiesthesia, Kirlian photography, and phototherapy, though undeniably based on using the measurements of "subtle energies" in both diagnosis and treatment, are so reliant on special equipment that they are not readily transferable into the clinics and offices where most of us go for help. Furthermore, these systems are to a large degree experimental and limited to a handful of researchers who are not readily available.

I share with Grossinger the feeling that whatever comes of research in the field of energy medicine, we may never be able to codify in acceptable terms the underlying principle behind the undoubted effectiveness of some of the energy therapies. In the meantime, just as Dr. Lewis Thomas has concluded that the earth cannot easily be conceived of as an "organism" because it is "too big, too complex, with too many parts lacking visible connections," so might we understand that the functions of the body also have "too many parts lacking visible connections." Yet even though the codifications of the workings of life energy may be ahead of us, or impossible, some systems are nevertheless available to us for integration into our present system of treatment and healing.

Structural Integration (Rolfing)

This system, developed by the late Ida Rolf, who was originally a biochemist in her native Switzerland, is a highly sophisticated, manipulative technique whereby a trained practitioner (known popularly as a "rolfer") attempts to change and align the physical structure of a human body in order to improve the physiological and psychological functioning of the person. This system developed out of Rolf's study of the effects of one of the most ⌄asic of all energies: gravitational force. Rolf came to believe that a body's relation to this ubiquitous force, which roots us all to the earth and which we universally take for granted, profoundly influences the vitality and well-being of human beings. She reasoned that as human beings evolved in the gravitational field of the earth, they developed a general structure, a muscular system, and a physiology to relate to this energy field. She further observed that the ideal relation between an upright human being and this universal force was a straight, vertical plane:

> For man is an energy field, as the earth in its outward envelope of forces is an energy field. How well a man can exist and function depends on whether the field that is himself, his psychological and physical personality, is reinforced or disorganized by the field of gravity. Looked at from this angle, gravity not only upholds a man, it feeds him. In a real and material world, this supporting energy can be supplied only as certain conditions are met. Gravity as a force acts as if it operated through a vertical, straight line at right angles to the Earth. Therefore, to profit from this flow, a man must be so organized that he operates as though he existed symmetrically around such a gravity line.

To achieve this ideal relationship between a human body and the gravitational force, the rolfer, through a vigorous massage of the deep fascia—the fibrous tissue between muscles that also forms the sheaths of the muscles and that envelops other deep, definitive structures like nerves or blood vessels—strives to correct the deviations from the vertical alignment of all the structural segments of the body: the head, the thorax, the pelvis, and the legs. The theory behind this manipulation is that the chemical and physical nature of the collagen fibers in fascial tissue allows the elasticity and resilience of the connective tissue to be changed. (Collagen is the albuminlike substance of the white fibers of connective tissues, cartilage, and bone.) The capacity of fascia to be stretched, then, allows for the realignment of the plastic structure of the body so that the goal of Structural Integration—the support of the energy field of man by the energy field of gravity—can be realized.

The causes for the deviation from the ideal vertical plane in which a straight line could be drawn through the ear, the shoulder, the hipbone, the knee, and the external shinbone of the ankle may be any one traumatic experience or a combination of such experiences. Physical accidents like knee injuries, for example, often cause displacements of bone and muscle that result in compensations that cause the pelvis and spine to rotate off the normal axis, or create a forward displacement of the head and neck in order to balance the body. Likewise, such structural deviations can have an emotional origin. Here Ida Rolf joins Wilhelm Reich, F. Matthias Alexander, Moshe Feldenkrais, and many other Western theorists about body-mind relationships in emphasizing the correspondence of the patterns of emotional and physical habits. All of them believe that human beings often "carry" their bodies in attitudes that manifest outwardly the inner feeling of, for example, fear, grief, or anger. The body becomes the stage on which is played out the emotional script, and if such a dramatization is allowed to persist in the muscular pattern of contraction, or shortening or thickening, then the material form of the drama— the muscle pattern—becomes involuntary and invariable. The cycle continues, then, as the fixed setting of the muscles establishes the emotional pattern in an equally rigid form. As the physical flesh, molded permanently, as it were, into a picture of the original emotional tone, "hardens" into constriction and restriction, the whole body becomes incapable of free flow and expression, with the result that the entire organism is fixed in one attitude, incapable of the full expression of either the normal emotional spectrum or the natural free range of the body.

Rolfing breaks into this endless cycle of emotional-physical relationship by applying strong mechanical energy to the body, attempting to release the connective tissue, reorganize the muscle relationships, and balance the body according to the defined norm of vertical alignment with the gravitational field.

The rolfing treatment itself is a series of ten one-hour manipulations which unwind and free the muscles, adjust the habitual compensations, and attempt to integrate and align the total structure. The technique differs from other massage and body manipulations in many ways. The pressure, kneading, and rubbing of the muscles is deep, and sometimes painful, both at the level of neuromuscular tenderness and in the release of profound emotional feelings that are reflected in the constriction and tension of the muscles. It aims not at establishing good posture (which can often be maintained at the cost of severe muscle tension) but at establishing a normal structure, an efficient alignment, that is experienced as effortless, more relaxed, even "lighter." Successful rolfing results in the full, upright extension of the whole body (actual increases in height measurements of people that have been rolfed have been recorded) and a symmetrical balancing of the body on both the left and right sides, the front and the back, the upper and lower parts of the body, resulting in a "lift" of the body and an increased gracefulness in free movement.

The release of muscle tension and the realignment of the segments of the body structure achieved through rolfing are believed to achieve many of the same effects on the personality and behavior as the practice of Hatha Yoga. Both systems are based on the belief that form influences consciousness, that psychological organization and biological organization are complementary parts of the human organism, that the body can be refined (if not materially redesigned) for the purpose of furthering psychological progress and growth. Like the *mudras* and *asanas* and rhythmic breathing processes of Yogic practice, the deep manipulation of the body through rolfing can affect human consciousness and enhance the possibility for expanded freedom and energy in the behavior of the total personality.

Therapeutic Touch

Dolores Krieger is a robust, energetic woman who is a professor in the Division of Nursing of the School of Education at New York University. She has been a nurse for many years, and also received her Ph.D. in education. Her personal style combines the gentle and caring approach we like to associate with efficient and considerate nurturing healers and the clear, tough-minded attitude of the true scholar.

In the late 1960s she became acutely conscious of the effects of increasing specialization in medicine, based as it was on what she saw as a reductionist view of human nature. She was captivated by the idea that only by addressing the totality of the human patient could true healing occur. Increasingly, she came to believe that there is inherent in all human beings an energy that facilitates healing in others. This point was dramatized for her when, in her job as a nurse, she participated in an experiment involving a world-renowned healer named Oskar Estebany, who treated patients with what, up to that time, had been called the "laying on of hands." This ancient practice has been reported as being common even four centuries before Christ, and is alluded to not only by early Greek writers but in documents like the Ebers Papyrus (see Chap. 4), which describes an Egyptian medical treatment dating back to 1552 B.C. that conforms to the traditional laying on of hands. Certainly in the beginning of the Christian era the technique was as central to religious practice as prayer and the administering of the sacraments. When the Christian church abandoned the practice, it was adopted by several kings of France and became known as the "royal touch."

Not until the late eighteenth century, however, was the scientific community ever involved in examining the dynamics of healing by touching. But when Franz Anton Mesmer made insistent, public claims that a "magnetic fluid" emanating from the human body was the mechanism of healing in the practice of the laying on of hands, the king of France appointed a commission to investigate Mesmer's assertions. That commission decided that Mesmer was wrong, and that the beneficial effects of the technique were due merely to "sensitive excitement, imagination, and imitation." Even though another French medical commission, which convened to repeat that investigation forty-seven years later, concurred with Mesmer's description of the "magnetic fluid," the idea of healing energy being transferred from one person to another remained a religious or folkloric notion for over one hundred years.

Oskar Estebany claimed that for at least ten years prior to his coming to the United States from his native Brazil, he had been curing patients with nothing more than his version of the old practice. This was especially dramatic inasmuch as the people Estebany had worked with were, for the most part, "end of the line" patients—that is, they had chronic illnesses that for many years had not improved as a result of conventional medical treatment.

Dolores Krieger marveled at the simplicity of Estebany's treatment. He sat quietly with patients, talked to them in a relaxed and friendly way, and literally laid his hands on them for fifteen or twenty minutes. The number of visits ranged from one to a dozen, and although the treatment never varied, the results were that a surprising number were found who had been improved considerably, and in some cases they were apparently cured of their chronic conditions.

There was nothing in Krieger's experience or training to explain this phenomenon, so she turned to a study of the literature on touching, in which she found little relating to this most fundamental of all human experiences. The most provocative and definitive work had been done, she found, by Dr. Bernard Grad at McGill University in the late 1950s and early 1960s, again working with Estebany. The subjects of his experiments were not human patients, but mice and plants. In the case of the mice, they were either "wounded" by surgically removing a patch of skin on their backs, or, in another case, given an iodine-deficient diet calculated to make them goitrous. In both groups, against which, of course, control groups of mice were measured, the effects of the laying on of Estebany's hands (either directly through holding the mice or indirectly through the holding of wool and cotton cuttings in which the mice lay in their cages) were significantly beneficial. The "wounded" mice in the Estebany group healed significantly faster than two other control groups, one treated by medical students and the other untreated. In the case of the mice fed a goitrogenic diet, the thyroids of those treated by Estebany increased in size significantly more slowly, and when the mice were returned to a normal diet, the goiters of those treated by the healer returned more quickly to normal than the mice in the other two groups. The same pattern of "healing" occurred when Estebany treated barley seeds that had been made "sick" with a saline solution. After five days it was discovered that the plants irrigated with water from flasks held by Estebany (as contrasted with those "treated" with water held by medical students) sprouted earlier, grew taller, and contained more chlorophyll.

Krieger found related experimental studies on enzyme levels, conducted by a biochemist nun, Sister M. Justa Smith. Again working with Estebany and other healers, Sister Justa concluded that the overall affects of the laying on of hands by healers contributed to the improvement or maintenance of general health.

From her study of these experiments, Krieger felt reinforced in her conviction that the human being is an open system, a crossroads for activity at many levels—physical, psychic, spiritual, organic, and inorganic—and, as such, is "exquisitely sensitive to wave phenomena, i.e., energy." To test this idea further Krieger did her own studies, choosing to go beyond wound repair and enzyme activity to look at hemoglobin values, one of the basic, systematic indices of the entirety of the body's basic metabolism. (Heme is one of the porphyrins, a basic source of energy in all living systems. It serves three major functions: the transport of oxygen, through which it supports the basis of body metabolism; electron transport, through which it carries an electric charge believed to accompany the healing of tissue; and heme acts as one of the detoxifiers of a number of compounds in the liver, the adrenal cortex, the lungs, and the placenta.) Patterning her own work after her observation of Estebany, and his experiments with Grad and Smith, Krieger developed her system, which she calls "therapeutic touch," which she is quick to acknowledge is merely a latter-day version of the traditional laying on of hands. (She sometimes laughingly says that she devised the term "therapeutic touch" simply because it is more palatable to "curriculum committees and other institutional bulwarks of modern society," but insists that her system is the same "personalized interaction" that occurs in the laying on of hands.)

Dolores Krieger believes that the power to transfer healing energy through touch, or sometimes merely by putting hands *near* the affected parts of a patient, is potential in all human beings. But she has always been quick and firm to say that the process is not merely "tender, loving care." To her the potential power can be actualized in those who themselves have "a fairly healthy body, a strong intent to help or heal ill persons, and who are educable." Her stipulations are based on the fact that as she has studied ancient medical systems such as acupuncture and Yogic therapy which proceed from a keystone belief in "energy flow" in the organism, she has come to identify the "fairly healthy person" as one who can be said to have an overabundance of *prana* (see Chap. 3), or *ch'i* (see Chap. 2), and that the resonance created by transferring that energy to a patient will act to reestablish the flow of *prana* or *ch'i*, enabling a person (if the system is not already too fragmented from chronic disease) to marshal that energy in the service of self-healing. She further realized that the touch involved in this process was not merely physiological, but rather a trained, humanized touch which itself conveyed the practitioner's *intent* to help or heal. At one point Krieger wrote, "Love itself, I found, is not enough to be truly therapeutic; you have to understand what you are doing, you have to act knowledgeably."

As of this writing, over ten thousand people have received training in therapeutic touch. They have come from every specialty and subspecialty in medicine and nursing, and there are thousands of others from other helping professions such as social work, psychotherapy, and the clergy, as well as laypersons from every walk of life. Therapeutic touch has been integrated into the preoperative and postoperative procedures in many surgical units and is used as a standard component of treatment in dozens of orthopedic, dental, chiropractic, and other therapeutic settings. Studies by Dr. Robert Swearingen, incidentally, have shown a decreased need for analgesic in orthopedic procedures through the use of therapeutic touch, and other studies have suggested strongly that post-surgical bleeding, the rate of recovery from surgery, and the subjective experience of pain are all significantly affected by the use of therapeutic touch as a regular part of treatment.

The implications of the future use of therapeutic touch are profound, both in the suggestive evidence of its direct use and because it is a model of how newly discovered techniques, often based on ancient theory or practice, may become integrated as adjunctive, complementary therapies in a broader and more humane medical encounter.

Chiropractic

Of the twenty-five thousand or so chiropractors in the United States, few would identify their therapy as a version of the "energy medicines" as we have defined the term. Most prefer to cite the historical evidence that chiropractic techniques are described in ancient Egyptian manuscripts, and that there is comparable documentary evidence that the ancient Hindus, Chinese, Babylonians, and Assyrians used manipulative techniques remarkably like the procedures employed by the modern practitioner. (The word "chiropratic" itself comes from two Greek words: *cheir*, "hand," and *praktikos*, "done by.")

But those same practitioners acknowledge that ancient forms of hand manipulation of the body to treat pain and disease have no historical continuity, and for all practical purposes disappeared as a formal method of therapy until 1895, when a Canadian named Daniel David Palmer performed a manipulation on the neck of the janitor in his office building, Harvey Lillard. Lillard had been deaf for seventeen years, "could not hear the racket of a wagon in the street, or the ticking of a watch." But Palmer, who had previously been a healer employing techniques of mesmerism (the precursor of modern hypnotherapy) had come to believe in a "universal intelligence" in all living matter, an intelligence that was ultimately responsible for the very existence, survival, and growth of all living organisms. Palmer concluded that in human beings the governing control mechanism was the nervous system, and he became convinced that human health was dependent on the unimpeded functioning of that system. Palmer believed that if the transmission of nervous impulses—such as those which make hearing possible—were blocked, the cause of the blockage was the mechanical impingement of nervous tissue secondary to what he called a "subluxation." A luxation, in conventional medical ter-

minology, is simply a dislocation, usually of a joint. By extension, a subluxation is an incomplete or partial dislocation, but Palmer's concern was
primarily with the spine, so his use of the term "subluxation" applied to
the thirty-one pairs of spinal nerves that travel down the spine from the
brain through a series of openings in the vertebrae, and was meant to
describe a condition where the partial loss of juxtaposition of one vertebra with the one above or below it, results both in an obstruction of the
opening between them and an impingement on surrounding nerves that
interferes with normal neurological functioning. So when Palmer
manipulated the specific vertebrae in the neck of Harvey Lillard, he did so
with the intent to realign the vertebrae of Lillard's spine and restore the
neurological process that enabled Lillard to "hear as before." Today chiropractic remains *primarily* concerned with the examination, diagnosis, and
treatment of the spine. Modern techniques of X-ray and other laboratory
procedures have been added to the basic, meticulous physical examination of the spine for subluxations, and just as their conventional medical
counterparts do, the modern chiropractors include dietary advice, exercise
regimes, nutritional supplements, and counseling on the details of
"healthy lifestyle habits" in their encounters with patients. These contemporary chiropractors associate themselves with the general tenets of
holistic health, sharing with other disciplines a conviction that preventive
techniques are to be favored over therapeutics in the long run, and the
tacit but firm belief in the inner healing power of the human body (Palmer's "universal intelligence," perhaps!)

To the degree that chiropractors join forces with holistic practitioners, they compound the continuing problem they have faced ever since
Dr. Palmer first treated Mr. Lillard—the controversy surrounding the efficacy of chiropractic and the corollary issue of outright disparagement by
the forces of conventional, scientific medicine. That battle has continued
for over eighty years, based on the position of the medical establishment
that the "single cause, single treatment" strategy of classical chiropractic
is primitive, unscientific, and dangerous. Until quite recently the standard
medical opinion of chiropractic was that by apparently ignoring the processes by which organs and tissues relax and contract *without* direct nervous stimulation—and still become diseased or damaged—the chiropractic manipulation of the spine to treat patients is at best simplistic, and at
worst, dangerous.

Historically, the antipathy of conventional physicians toward chiropractic took the form of ostracism and powerful legislative lobbying
aimed at keeping chiropractic outside the consensual health care system,
thereby implying that patients took the same uninformed risk with the
chiropractor that they ran by going to a faith healer, a magician or other
"fringe" practitioner to seek relief and cure. But the word-of-mouth anecdotal reports of patients who persisted in using chiropractors, together
with the persistence and more sophisticated organization of chiropractors

as a professional group, kept the field alive, and as increasing studies in the United States, Canada, and New Zealand of chiropractic effectiveness have seemed to confirm its usefulness, the war between the medical establishment and chiropractic has waned dramatically. Today the some seventeen hundred annual graduates of thirteen accredited chiropractic colleges not only find adequate numbers of patients to fill their practice, but they are legally licensed in all fifty states, and their services are covered by Medicare health insurance, Medicaid programs, and an increasing number of union and other private health insurance plans. It has been estimated that anywhere from 3.5 to 35 *million* Americans use chiropractic regularly, either as their only therapeutic resource or as an adjunct to orthodox medical care.

Today, with chiropractic so firmly established in its own right (three new chiropractic colleges are in formation at this writing), the issue is not chiropractic versus medicine, but rather where chiropractic fits in an enlarged map of the health care system. There is still argument that chiropractic is too narrow, both in theory and technique, to be used as a form of primary medical care. The expanding curriculum in chiropractic training (students are required to have two years of college before spending four Western-science-oriented years in chiropractic college) is aimed at giving chiropractic graduates a much richer training in nutrition, physiology, biochemistry, and other biomedical subjects than they have traditionally received. But even sympathetic orthodox medical practitioners still believe that chiropractic should confine itself to manipulation for spine-related disorders and not attempt to compete as an alternative, comprehensive approach to health care.

Palmer himself preached against drugs (and even natural medicines like herbs) and the water cures and electrical therapies of his day because they were palliative instead of curative, a charge that lies at the heart of much of the resistance to orthodox medicine today. Moreover, since chiropractic is dominantly characterized by hands-on contact with the patient in an extremely personal and often informal environment, the modern chiropractor is often a model of the caring, humanistic, collegial healer who provides the humane and nurturing attention that many of us find lacking in the authoritarian, technology-bound physician we meet so often.

Applied Kinesiology

One of the most provocative latter-day developments to emerge from chiropractic is the diagnostic technique known as applied kinesiology. "Kinesiology" is the generic term meaning the science of the anatomy, physiology, and mechanics of purposeful movement in human beings. "Applied kinesiology" is the name coined by Dr. George J.

Goodheart, who reasoned that the subluxation of one or more vertebrae could obviously interfere with normal muscular function, and that in addition to the use of spinal X-ray examination, the observation and palpation of bones and tissues involved in posture and movement, the measurements of arm and leg length, the analysis of skin temperature, and the overall analysis of posture—all of which are used at one time or another in chiropractic diagnosis—the specific testing of muscles could reveal the need for chiropractic manipulation and lead the practitioner directly to the offending vertebra. Goodheart's technique of muscle testing, however, is not merely the conventional feeling for spasm, tightness, or simple weakness. His method is based on a specific theory that *weak muscles on one side of the body can cause normal opposing muscles to become tight.* Kinesiologists liken the principle to the effect of a door being held in place by two springs so that it can swing either way: As long as the tension on both springs is equal, the door remains in place (the "system is in balance"). If the spring on either side of the door weakens, the opposite spring immediately becomes knotted in taking up the slack. Lubricating the knotted spring will not restore the mechanical imbalance. Only by replacing or strengthening the weak spring can the balance be restored.

The action of the two springs is a metaphor for most muscular activity in the human body. For every motion a muscle makes, there is a corresponding muscle which *opposes* that motion. There are muscles which extend the legs, arms, hands, and feet—and their opposite numbers which contract those same body parts. Since muscles move not only back and forth in the same line, there are others that perform the function of pronating, or rotating. Again, there are two sets for each possible motion, one to turn inward toward the midline of the body, another to perform the task of turning part of the body away from the midline.

Goodheart reasoned that if the tight muscle—identified by spasm or the subjective experience of pain or "knot"—is one which flexes, say, the arm of the patient, one could reasonably expect to find weakness in the muscle that extends or straightens that arm. If a tight muscle pulls a limb *away* from the body, Goodheart looked for a muscle which pulls the limb in to be weak—and so on, for all the motions the human body can make with up to forty-two major muscle pairs.

Applied kinesiology, then, provides the diagnosis of the precise muscle which will benefit from treatment. In this instance, since Goodheart was a chiropractor, the treatment of choice was, of course, manipulation of the identified muscle or of the spinal vertebra associated with that muscle. Over the twenty years Goodheart has been teaching the principles of applied kinesiology, more and more chiropractors have adopted the system as an adjunct to the other, more classical diagnostic procedures of chiropractic. And as some chiropractors seek to become more holistic in their approach, giving advice on diet, nutritional supplements, exercise, and other aspects of what have come to be known as "lifestyle habits," some have extended the theory of applied kinesiology to the area of testing for allergic responses and other symptoms not usually associated with the postural and mechanical concerns of traditional chiropractic. This is especially true when, after the muscle-testing diagnosis has been completed and the appropriate manipulation applied, the original presenting symptoms have not been relieved. Applied kinesiology assumes that the weakness that has been treated can have as its root cause a specific, individual allergy in the patient and that the muscles can once again be "read" for weakness to determine the offending substance.

A typical test for allergy in applied kinesiology consists in taking a small amount of the suspect substance into the mouth and chewing, but not swallowing, it. The material may be one of the foods that has a widespread reputation for being an allergenic—strawberries, milk, or shellfish, for example—or it may be something like tobacco or a particular kind of alcoholic liquor, at which point a standard applied kinesiology muscle test is employed; if the muscle goes weak, the substance is identified as an allergen to the subject. A number of standard applied kinesiology muscle tests are used, but one of the most common involves the muscle known as the *opponens pollicis,* the chief muscle in the fatty mound of the thumb, and the *abductor minimi digiti,* the muscle that runs along the ulnar (outer) edge of the palm and that connects with the tendons of the little finger. In this test the subject touches the tip of the thumb to the tip of the little finger, forming a ring. The kinesiologist places a finger from each of his hands inside this ring, and tests the strength of the muscles by pulling the patient's thumb and little finger apart. A bit of separation on the test is considered normal, and if the muscles lock after being pulled apart a bit, they are considered strong. The test for allergy is done, of course, while the ingested but unswallowed substance is in the mouth, and the test results compared by patient and practitioner with the same test done prior to taking the suspect substance. A weaker performance with the substance in the mouth, of course, will lead to the recommendation that the patient forgo eating, drinking, or smoking the offending item.

In addition to testing for allergies, many applied kinesiologists have added nutritional advice to their armamentarium of treatments. Thus, in the instance of the test for weakness in the *opponens pollicis,* the practitioner may conclude that the demonstrated weakness may result in the syndrome known as "tennis elbow," and in addition to the manipulation of the related vertebrae and muscles may recommend that raw bone supplements be added to the diet, as well as food rich in calcium, such as milk and milk products, bone meal, and dolomite.

Applied kinesiology theory, in other words, has expanded not only the diagnostic approach of the modern chiropractor, but also the range of therapeutic maneuvers that are used in treatment. Since modern chiropractic is dedicated to the notion that the human body possesses an "innate intelligence," they now see their work as including any natural therapeutic approach that will relieve the blocks to that power and make possible a maintenance of health.

Touch for Health

Another system with its roots in chiropractic theory goes even farther in working on what it calls the "energy flow" in the human body. Touch for Health, which its developer, Dr. John F. Thie, calls "a new approach to restoring our natural energies," uses not only applied kinesiology techniques for testing and diagnosis, but also employs what Thie calls "acupressure touch" in treatment, a form of light acupressure, for working on the identified weak muscles. In addition, since Thie also had training in nutrition, his system includes dietary advice, though the emphasis is on working with the structural, mechanical aspects of the body —the entire musculoskeletal system.

Thie's attitude toward the classical meridians of Chinese medicine is unique. He refers to them as "acupuncture vessels," and believes they contain a free-flowing, colorless, "noncellular" liquid, which is activated, at least in part, by the heart. He points out that the meridians have been confirmed by measuring their radioactivity and electrical resistance and that the points along the meridians are electromagnetic in character. But he departs from most therapists in the field of Oriental medicine when he describes the energy flow along the meridians as a "liquid," claims that the points "consist of small, oval cells called bonham corpuscles," that these cells "surround the capillaries in the skin, the blood vessels in the organs throughout the body," and that there are five hundred such points in the human body.

Despite these theoretical differences in describing the energy flow, Touch for Health follows the other basic principles of Chinese medicine (see Chap. 2)—the theory of *yin* and *yang,* the concepts of "blocked" or "overactive" energy in the meridians, the law of the Five Elements, the law of mother-son, and the idea that the balancing of energy puts the body in the best possible condition to heal itself of ailments or maintain good health. (Of course, because of its link with chiropractic and applied kinesiology, Touch for Health emphasizes that spinal alignment, the correction of postural deviations and distortions, and muscle tone are the key signposts of good health.) In diagnosis Touch for Health substitutes muscle testing for the traditional reading of the pulses in Chinese medicine, and likewise substitutes hands and fingers for the classical acupuncture needles. In fact, Touch for Health prescribes testing one muscle associated with each of the fourteen meridians. If the muscle is strong, indicated by its locking and staying in place under the muscle test, it is assumed that there is at least enough energy flowing in that meridian to enable a muscle to function normally. If, on the other hand, the muscle is weak, meaning that it is shaky or inappropriately soft, or permits the arm or leg to give way under the test, it is assumed that the flow of energy in that meridian needs to be stimulated.

For example, in testing the Lung Meridian (which you may recall from Chap. 2 runs from the chest down the outside edge of the front of the arm, ending in the tip of the thumb) the associated muscle for testing is called the *anterior serratus* (the muscle that drives the shoulder blade forward and raises the ribs). In the Touch for Health muscle test, the patient either sits or stands with the arm held out straight at the shoulder level, angled about forty-five degrees from the side of the body, with the thumb up. The Touch for Health practitioner, holding the tip of the shoulder blade with one hand to prevent it from sliding down, uses the other hand and arm to exert pressure against the forearm of the patient, attempting to bring it down toward the floor. (See illustration.)

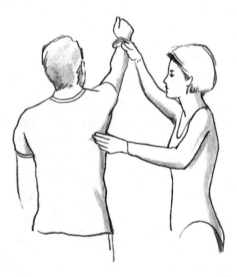

It is the resistance to this pressure, measured against the definitions of "strong" or "weak" mentioned above, that determines the "acupressure touch" points to be used in treatment. If the Touch for Health practitioner determines that the Lung Meridian needs strengthening ("stimulating" in Chinese medicine) he or she applies the "touch for health" to points on the hands and feet on the same side as the muscle that has been tested. Touch for Health acupressure technique is always done on two related points at one time, and if more than two points are specified, the Touch for Health manual, or a Touch for Health instructor in a training workshop, will indicate the order in which the points are treated. In the instance of strengthening the Lung Meridian, the first two points treated are Spleen-3, on the inner side of the sole of the foot at the middle of the first metatarsal bone (big toe). (See illustration.)

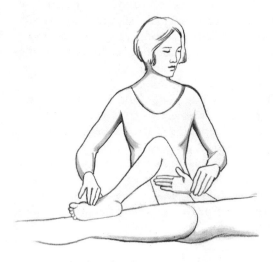

Simultaneously, the point pressed on the arm is Lung-9, the point on the wrist bone immediately below the fleshy ball of the thumb. The second set of points are on the hand only: Lung-10, the point on the palmar surface of the thumb at the middle of the first metacarpal bone, and Heart-8, the point lying on the outer edge of the hand just above the wrist crease. (See illustration.)

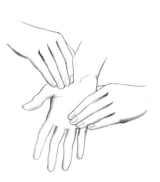

Touch for Health acupressure differs from traditional acupressure techniques as practiced by Chinese physicians. While the latter use fingertips, the pads of the fingers, or even the fingernails to apply pressure, depending on the condition being treated, and apply pressure while rotating the finger for up to three minutes on each set of points, Touch for Health uses "as many fingers on or around the point as will fit," applying light pressure for about thirty seconds. When working on the legs, Touch for Health practitioners are taught also to feel for a pulse of about seventy to seventy-four beats per minute as a sign that pressure is to be released. Touch for Health practitioners are aware that the technique does not insure precision as to specific point pressure, but are more interested in working with the meridians rather than the exact points that lie along them.

Again with regard to the Lung Meridian, if the *anterior serratus* muscle tests as tight or painful, or otherwise indicates a need for weakening, the Touch for Health therapist again applies pressure to pairs of points, in this case first to Kidney-10, on the inner side of the leg halfway around from the kneecap, and Lung-5, in the crook of the elbow at the outside front edge of the arm, and then again to Lung-10 and Heart-8. There is no difference in the pressure technique between strengthening or weakening, only a difference in the points to be manipulated. (Note that the second set of points is the same for strengthening or weakening the lung meridian.)

In a complete Touch for Health examination and treatment, the process of testing and "holding," as Touch for Health people sometimes call an acupressure technique, is repeated for all forty-two of the muscle pairs that are central to chiropractic and kinesiology theory. The treatment is pleasant and gentle, and throughout their work, the Touch for Health practitioners emphasize the caring and loving nature of touch in general. And even though the prime goal in the Touch for Health approach is "spinal integrity" or "postural correctness," it remains true that through this amalgam of Oriental and Western ideas of whole health, Touch for Health practitioners have not only provided relief from pain and disability of many kinds, but have been successful, too, in helping people maintain an improved level of overall health.

Shiatsu

The dominant massage system in the Western world for the past two hundred years has been the so-called "Swedish" or "medical" massage. The familiar vigorous rubbing and kneading of the muscles, developed in Western Europe alongside plastic surgery and therapeutic calisthenics, is now a formally acknowledged component of the medical subspecialty known as physical therapy, applied not only for purposes of rehabilitation and strengthening of the body after trauma, but also as a preventive or supportive practice for active people.

In the East massage has an even older history, having been one of the four arms of classical Chinese medicine ever since the mapping of the energy meridians (called *keiraku* in Japanese). Along with the practice of T'ai Chi and other exercise systems, massage as a form of physiotherapy has been taught for thousands of years in both the formal, academic schooling of Chinese physicians and the "tribal" or oral tradition passed on from master to apprentice through the centuries.

At almost the same time the Chinese acupuncture theory and practice was adopted in Japan, a variation of the complex, rhythmical *amma* massage from China began to develop, until in the middle of this century the formal system called Shiatsu *(shi,* "finger," and *atsu,* "pressure") became legally sanctioned in Japan, alongside the *amma* and the Western style of massage.

Shiatsu is a more localized system than the other two, being essentially the strong, direct, perpendicular application of pressure to the acupuncture points located along the meridians through which *ki* (the Japanese term for the *ch'i* energy of Chinese medicine) flows in an unending cycle. In the same way that the needles of acupuncture are used to tonify or sedate this energy so as to bring the body into balance, so Shiatsu works toward the same end, but using fingers and pressure instead of needles to achieve the desired changes. In Shiatsu the points along the meridians—of which the Shiatsu practitioner uses about 92 of the 360 standard locations—are called *tsubos,* and the practitioner leans on these points with considerable weight in the Shiatsu treatment. The heart of Shiatsu strategy is the principle that prolonged pressure is required. Some theorists believe that through this deep and extended pressure the effect works on the parasympathetic nervous system, which tends to retard circulation, and by pressing hard and long, the effect is a deeper state of relaxation of both the mind and the body. Generally, the practitioner uses both hands at all times, pressing on two points at a time in an effort to balance the flow of energy along the entire course of the meridian. The thumbs are the chief instruments of pressure, as they are generally the strongest of the hand's digits, but the index, middle, and ring fingers are also used for some treatments. Occasionally, the palm or even the elbow is used as well. The ball of the thumb and fingers are pushed, never the tip, and the strong pressure is applied evenly for five to seven seconds, except in the sensitive neck area, where only three seconds of pressure is used. (Shiatsu practitioners are always careful to keep their fingernails cut short and to warm their hands before working on patients.) As in standard Chinese acupressure the patient should feel a sensation somewhere between pleasure and pain. This is particularly relevant in Shiatsu, in which the technique calls for the practitioner to apply the weight of his whole body to the pressure on the patient. The Shiatsu therapist prepares himself quite carefully before the treatment. In addition to making sure the room in which he is working is kept clean, quiet, and warm, he does not begin work until the patient is relatively relaxed. Some Shiatsu practitioners work on standard massage tables, but most prefer to use exercise mats or a well-carpeted floor. When working on the back, the patient lies flat on his stomach with his face turned sideways (with no pillow under the head), his arms at his sides, and his rib cage as flat and evenly distributed as possible. When the stomach and the front of the body are being worked on, the patient lies on his back, with his arms at his sides, and with a small pillow under his head. In both positions he is encouraged to keep his mouth slightly open and his eyes closed.

Shiatsu pressure is applied only when the patient is exhaling, so the therapist pays close attention to the patient's—and his own—breathing rhythm. As orthopedists and chiropractors would agree, the body becomes harder and tighter during the inhalation cycle of breathing, and pressure applied at that time might cause discomfort, or even muscle spasms. Treatments generally last between thirty minutes and one hour, and the patient is urged to rest for a short period when it has been completed. Throughout, the patient is urged to inhale and exhale in a relaxed and regular pattern, to give in as completely as possible to the therapeutic pressure.

Shiatsu is usually used in two forms: For general health maintenance, or the prevention of stress during a particularly trying time of life, a general Shiatsu massage of the entire body is employed. As a curative technique for common ailments ranging from asthma to toothache, short treatments to specific points may be used and repeated as needed until relief is experienced. (Many of the acupressure techniques described in Part II of this book are adapted from Shiatsu practice.)

The serious Shiatsu practitioners are quite modest in their claims and goals. They consider the main purpose of the technique to be the relief of symptoms, or help in recovering from the fatigue and strain of everyday life, rather than as a cure for chronic disease. They do not treat people with contagious diseases or with any disorder of the heart, liver, kidney, or lungs, or with cancer, sarcoma, or infectious skin diseases. Shiatsu is never given when the patient is either very hungry or before two hours after eating a big meal. Nor would a Shiatsu treatment be indicated if a patient is very tired, sweating heavily, or has a fast heartbeat. In these instances the Shiatsu practitioner might wait awhile to see if these conditions return to normal and would proceed with treatment if they did.

One of the American embellishments on the traditional Shiatsu system that is popularly talked about is the technique of walking over the patient's body, and, indeed, if the practitioner knows the patient well, he may gently tread over the spine, arms, and legs of his patient to expand the effect of having worked on specific *tsubos*. When done properly this form of treatment is surprisingly pleasurable and adds to the overall sense of well-being that usually follows a Shiatsu session.

But the standard hands-only massage of Shiatsu is usually quite enough to benefit the patient. When the technique is done well it can go a long way toward awakening the inherent strengths and balances of the body, and even for the truly cynical a good Shiatsu massage can create a communal sense between the toucher and the touched that makes it easier to believe that the harmony of vital energy fields is indeed a defining characteristic of true health.

Most conventionally trained physicians either laugh or sneer at these therapies (or warn of the dangers of their sometimes extreme manipulations), acknowledging only that the alleged benefits derived from them may be due to such nonscientific causes as placebo or hypnotic effects, or because the various manipulations accidentally make successful adjustments of the distorted anatomy or physiology of a disabled body. On the other hand, many of the impassioned practitioners of these therapies claim that their systems are comprehensive enough to treat not only neuromuscular disorders but also most of what ails the vulnerable human body, and can be employed without dependence on the medications and procedures of conventional medicine.

This debate, of course, is between people who rarely communicate directly with each other or attempt seriously to learn either the philosophy or the technical practices of those they oppose. The difference is that one camp—orthodox medical practice—is politically and economically in charge of mainstream medical service and, for the most part, does not open its doors to any of the energy medicines, even as adjunctive therapies. As a result, we see a whole array of manipulative systems functioning competitively outside the consensual system. As of this writing, that community of alternative therapists is, in effect, a group of new "specialists," somewhat comparable to the radiologists, neurologists, psychiatrists, and surgeons who are comfortably ensconced within conventional medical institutions. But where family physicians, pediatricians, or general internists confidently make referrals to specialists with similar educational backgrounds, they almost never make use of the resources of the energy specialists, whose work they neither acknowledge or understand. These outsiders survive largely on the word-of-mouth referrals of former patients and colleagues in their own field.

This situation is prolonged, of course, by the sometimes excessive and often strident claims of the practitioners of the energy medicines, bent as they seem to be on demonstrating that their systems offer *more* complete healing methods than conventional, scientific medicine. So they, too, add to the confusion and fear that besets the patient who is seeking help when classical therapies have failed to effect a cure, or relief from pain.

In the case of chiropractic, some measure of communication is beginning to take place. In what has been called "probably the most comprehensive and detailed independent examination of chiropractic ever undertaken in any country," an official commission of inquiry in New Zealand concluded that "modern chiropractic is far from being an 'unscientific cult' . . . is safe . . . can be effective in relieving musculo-skeletal symptoms. . . . Chiropractors should, in the public interest, be accepted as partners in the general health care system. . . ." This report has led to a wide-ranging discussion in the American medical press, and some American physicians are now calling for the professional integration described in the New Zealand report, albeit with chiropractors assuming a "limited" role in the overall scheme of medical service, something like the status now granted to speech therapists, dentists, podiatrists, optometrists, and so on. Proponents of this synthesis also cite the circumstances in Canada, where chiropractic is routinely reimbursed under a socialized medical system, and where hostility between medical doctors and chiropractors is minimal. To all this has been added increasing public exposure of the active part played by many chiropractors in the training and treatment of well-known athletes, demonstrating on a broad scale the surprisingly general belief that chiropractic manipulation is helpful.

But this dialogue, like many of the interdisciplinary discussions of acupuncture, does not signal an emerging rapport at the theoretical level. Even those physicians who advocate opening the medical establishment to practitioners of Chinese medicine or chiropractic neither comprehend nor accept the ideas about energy that underlie such therapies. Rather, the accommodation, when it occurs, is founded on a somewhat grudging admission that beneficial results derive from these therapeutic techniques and that on this ground of efficacy these systems should be at least partially officialized.

Indeed, that pragmatic evaluation may be all we are capable of dealing with at this point. It is clearly not necessary for either the provider or the patient to fully understand or believe in the theory of energy manipulation in order for the technique to be helpful. Apart from the common emphasis on knowledgeable and caring touch, what may be occurring, in fact, is that all of the systems described above, and others such as polarity therapy, cranial manipulation, zone therapy, Do-in, Lomi therapy, the Alexander technique, etc., are simply different ways of dealing with stress reactions in the body, and that when they succeed, they do so because they help the patient increase the awareness of the inevitable mind-body-emotions connection, and in so doing, imply the increased control that may be learned from professional treatment and self-care.

As Nikolaas Tinbergen put it in his Nobel Prize acceptance speech in 1973, "It need not cause surprise that a mere gentle handling of body muscles can have such profound effects on both body and mind. The more that is being discovered about psychosomatic diseases, and in general about the complex two-way traffic between the brain and the rest of the body, the more obvious it has become that too rigid a distinction between mind and body is of only limited use to medical science, in fact can be a hindrance to its advance."

I went not only to the doctors, but also to barbers, bathkeepers, learned physicians, women, and magicians who pursue the art of healing; I went to alchemists, monasteries, to nobles and the common folk, to the experts and the simple.

Paracelsus (1493–1541)

7.
GRANDMOTHER MEDICINE:
Remedies of Improvisation and Hearsay

All medicine is folk medicine. The aspirin or Valium tablet, the birth control pill, and the decongestant spray are as much reflections of modern culture and civilization as were the garlic bulb, the lemon juice, and the clay of countless "primitive" societies that preceded ours. Medicine, like music and painting and language, arises as an expression of human ingenuity in response either to the external world or the stirrings of the soul; the theories or practices of medicine are usually defined by the dominant worldview of a time and place.

Medicine, of course, stands apart from the arts in one vital respect: Its intention is utilitarian, focused on the goal of the relief of pain and the preservation of life. Not for medicine the sportive pleasures of philosophical speculation that need not arrive at an answer, but that gives its pleasures in the endless examination of the question. Not for medicine the effects of music or poetry or painting, which often present us the vision of better worlds, images of the possibilities as well as the tragedies of being human. Most medicine is, by definition, remedial and immediate, practical and serious, concrete and realistic. If all medicine is folk medicine, it is also emergency medicine, claiming an insistent priority over the indulgences of art, the pursuit of profit or comfort, or the pleasures of inactivity.

So medicine emerges from more than the simple stretching of human imagination and invention; its roots are in the urgency of accidents and injuries, the wounds of enemy stones and arrows, the assault of hostile weather, the attacks of frightened, vicious animals. In short, all external threats to survival demand medicine, the word derived from the Indo-European root, *med-* which, as Guido Majno says, "seems to imply the general connotation of 'thoughtful action to establish order,'" an interpretation reflected in many of the words descended from the same root: "median," "meditate," "measure," and the word "remedy" itself.

In whatever language we use, a remedy is still defined as "anything used in the treatment of disease." A remedy need not work—that is, make a positive change in the condition for which it is employed—and it certainly need not be consistent with time or culture. A remedy need not be a substance at all, as we know from modern psychotherapy and its antecedents in the rituals of shamans, sorcerers, magicians, and priests. And a remedy need not derive from an organized or a rationalized theory, nor be applied by a designated practitioner schooled in religious or scientific notions about healing. Human touch, simply human presence, has as honorable a history of benefitting the ill as incantations or medications.

The comparison of relatively primitive remedies of old folk medicine with the sophisticated therapies of a computer age does an injustice to both. Such a comparison, on the one hand, leads us to the wholesale rejection of all that is old or uncomplicated or informal; or on the other hand, to the blanket distrust of all that is new or complex or highly organized. In following that line of reasoning we repeat the age-old conflict between the empirical and the rational schools of medicine that has been so well documented by scholars. (See particularly Harris Coulter and Richard Grossinger.) They point out that from the earliest times (at least in Europe, since the Assyrians, the Egyptians, the Hindus, and the Chinese seem not to have been so divided), the two perspectives on health and illness have been at odds. The empiricist believed, and believes, in the idiosyncrasy and uniqueness of every symptom and each individual person, and moves from one discrete situation to another, applying remedies from a storehouse of experience, but selecting such remedies based on the unique and detailed qualities of the illness he observes, and as it is described by the ailing person. He disdains the abstract and theoretical knowledge derived from the organized study of the chemical (physiological) and mechanical (anatomical) behavior of cadavers or diseased bodies. From his own experience with pathological conditions in living patients he selects from his armamentarium of therapies the one he has seen work curatively before. The rationalist, on the other hand, seeks to generalize the laws of healing. To achieve this he studies the etiology (the origin and "natural" course) of disease processes, and his intent is especially focused on the application of a quick, mechanical treatment of a dominant, single symptom he has identified. The rationalist may have some concern with the many layers of the total organismic involvement with distress, but his emphasis is clearly on applying an immediate remedy that squares with his commitment to the concrete theory of cause and effect.

In modern, organized, consensual medicine—the medicine increasingly paid for, monitored, and managed by governments in an unsettled partnership with corporations—the rationalist view has clearly triumphed. The development of the science of medicine has paralleled, and to some extent has been modelled on, the comparable development of modern physics and chemistry, and the highly technologized care of hospital patients is the prime example of the union of all three in their most sophisticated forms. The well-known CAT scans (computerized axial tomography) used in identifying the details of inner pathology, and the use of lasers and radioactive iodine in disease management, are examples of the way physics, chemistry, and medicine have merged to form the modern version of the rationalist approach to disease and disability. And the sophisticated laboratory techniques of the rationalists have often validated the remedies of the empirical school, leading to at least the limited integration of ancient remedies into the current single, scientific practice of medicine. As Erwin Ackerknecht wrote, "It is amazing what an enormous number of effective drugs is known to the primitives. From 25 to 50 percent of their pharmacopoeia is often found to be objectively active. Our knowledge of opium, hashish, hemp, coca, cinchona, eucalyptus, sarsaparilla, acacia, kousso, copaibo, guiac, jolep, podophyllin, quessic, and many others is a heritage from the primitive."

So although the rationalist viewpoint has become dominant in technical medicine, the empirical tradition has not disappeared. From the outset empiricism has been largely an oral tradition, passed on as part of the cultural and religious life of peoples all over the world. The empirical approach may not dominate the urban teaching hospitals in which health professionals get their training, but it survives everywhere, not just as anecdotal lore but at the heart of the medical systems used by millions of people all over the world who do not have access to what we consider mainstream medicine. In fact, in absolute numbers more people are treated by techniques that derive from the empirical tradition than are served by rationalist institutions.

In the beginning, of course, there was only medicine, the improvisational, idiosyncratic, local, and direct response to human distress. The only models for relieving such distress were provided by animals and the natural world. Man drew resin from trees to bind his wounds in imitation of the trees themselves, and he may well have learned from animals the lesson that all damaged tissue has almost miraculous regenerative powers. (We cannot be sure that human beings did not also learn many of the basic gestures of first aid from apes and chimpanzees, whose skill and delight in tending to injuries is well documented. For example, study of chimpanzee "grooming" behavior led researchers to find that more than hygiene and cosmetics are involved in many of the interactions of the animals. For instance, not only does a chimpanzee perform a helpful first aid maneuver to remove a foreign object from the eye, an animal so affected approaches another with a specific supplicatory movement *asking* for the help. Interestingly, the "practitioner" gives evidence of great pleasure after the successful "operation.") In other words, as Bruno Gebhardt has said, "medicine is older than the medical profession." What we now call "scientific medicine" is only the current chapter in a long history of the human race attempting to minister to its debilities.

Priests, Plants, and Panaceas

From what we know of that history, there appear to be three major strains to the folk medical efforts of our forebears. It seems clear that the first organized system addressed to healing was bound up with the inevitable religious practice of the ancients. In every antique culture a version of a shaman or priest caste was well defined. And though the distresses that demanded their attention may have been physical, the healing ritual and process was addressed to the spiritual plane of people's existence. From the *ashipu* of Egypt to the chanting medicine man of the Navajo, the designated tribal healer performed his word magic employing occult charms, formulas, spells, conjurations, and blessings that have been passed on to him through what we would call his "medical training." In almost all cases we see what he did as a blend of magic and rude knowledge, a synthesis of the rational and the ritual, with not a little of his effectiveness depending on psychological manipulation. After all, his powers and procedures were not confined to the treatment of purely physical complaints; many of the same things he did for fractures and fevers were employed, too, to deal with hexes, love affairs, capital improvement, crop growth, and the whole spectrum of universal human tribulations.

The shaman was generally presumed to be either the present incarnation of a previously powerful healer or saint, or have access to such a prior figure, or at least be able to call forth such a healer from the spirit world to participate in the healing treatment. If any single theme linked all the variations of the shaman/priest's role, it was a belief that the ancient and traditional held the key to knowledge and health—in sharp contrast to our modern assumption that "newer is better." Imbued with a mythic sense of totemism and a feeling of profound and perpetual closeness to brute nature, the shaman was at once a visionary and a natural healer, empirical in his attitude, spiritual in his practice, and deriving his power from the vision he shared with his tribe that the forces which had formed the natural world could be invoked to repair the accidents and afflictions that arose in that world. What set the shaman apart from others was that he worked in an organized way at communicating and merging with the forces of nature as the tribe conceived them, and through such efforts (and his own presumed good health) transmitted to the ill and the wounded, the cursed and the deprived, the strength they needed to recover and survive. And as Richard Grossinger has said, "We must not be misled by the primitivity of native medicine. Wisdom is there, experiment is there; only the awakened objective mind is not."

Tribal Medicine

The second theme we have derived historically from ancient cultures is what anthropologists have come to call "ethnomedicine" or "indigenous" medicine. It cannot be known how this strain of medical activity arose, since, after all, there is no reliable record of a "revolt" against shamanism, and, indeed, vestiges of the shamanic approach have not only survived, but there are countless people in both hemispheres still being healed by rituals and practices remarkably similar to what we believe were prehistoric traditions. Still, in many parts of the world a specific and local medical practice developed, based less on the consensual religious ideas about nature and the human body, and more on specific and intimate knowledge of regional substances—herbs, foodstuffs, or improved implements—that were used to treat afflictions of all kinds. The Ayurvedic medicine of ancient India (see Chap. 3) and the acupuncture, massage, and herbalism of Oriental medicine (see Chap. 2) are descendants of the regional or ethnic medicines that formed alongside the shamanic.

From the shamanic tradition these systems extracted, improved, and expanded the range of botanical prescriptions, but where the shaman would accompany medications with chanting or trance healing to exorcise the "evil spirits" causing internal distress, the indigenous local systems devised medical instruments to perform what we call surgery: making incisions, scratching or scarring the flesh, cutting into parts of the anatomy, including even the skull. (The procedure of trepanation, for example, an operation to remove a portion of the bone of the skull with stone or bronze tools, was commonly performed in prehistoric times in many cultures. The evidence of healing at the edges of such discovered bones suggests that the survival rate of patients who underwent this painful procedure was close to 100 percent!) But surgery was not the chief technique of the indigenous medicines that took root in primitive societies alongside shamanic healing. In Africa, Asia, Europe, and the Americas, other less severe mechanical procedures were widespread: Massage, bathing, sweat bathing, cupping (the application of very hot cups to bring blood to the skin's surface), superficial incisions, and bloodletting were employed throughout the world.

Even more important than manipulative procedures and the surgery of primitive medicine was the evolution and concerted expansion of pharmaceutical medicines, the dosing of patients with medications made from plants, animals (including reptiles, fish, and insects), rocks, minerals, chalk dust, ashes, charcoal, earth, and sand. By the time of the first century after Christ, Pliny the Elder could write, "Nature distributed medicines everywhere; even the very desert was made a drug store," knowing as he did from his studies and the reports of returning soldiers and travelers that not only in his own Roman culture, but on the coasts of Africa and in the mountain kingdoms of Asia the use of nature's bounty in the treatment of illness, disease, and accident was common. As noted, these medicines are the ancestors of the modern pharmacy, particularly along the historical line that runs from common plants to the modern synthetic compound. (The connection, for instance, that links the early use of the bark of the willow tree as a painkiller to the current dependence on aspirin for the same purpose is direct and clear-cut. In our ethnic arrogance and chauvinistic modernism we label the use of willow bark as "primitive" and the use of the aspirin tablet as "sophisticated," but even contemporary scientists must acknowledge that the essential ingredient that makes both effective is the same: salicin, which the body converts into salicylic acid. See Chaps. 4 and 5 for more specific examples of the genealogy of herbalism and modern pharmaceuticals.)

The accumulation of a vast botanical pharmacopoeia was not casual, and despite the international flavor of Pliny's observation about the universality of healing substances, the indigenous medicines of Asia, Europe, and the Americas were characterized by intensive experimentation with local materials. In contrast to modern clinical investigations, in which a new drug may be evaluated in a few days, primitive experimenters took decades to examine the effects of their medications. The initiation of boys into the profession as medicine men took place when they were adolescents, and their training in the curative powers of their region's substances continued throughout adult life. In the case of some North American Indian tribes, for instance, there arose what we would call "specialists," medicine men who were expert at treating one or two of the few diseases that befell the Native Americans before the coming of the white man. Everywhere the assumption was the same—"every tree, bush, and plant has a use"—and today Navajos recall that their grandfathers told them of the wisdom of the ancients: "If you should injure yourself when you are alone, hunting in the mountains, do not move; remain quiet, and look carefully around you—even if you have broken a limb you will find within your arm's reach a plant that has been placed there to help you relieve your pain." (The names of some known curative plants seem to have derived from both their common locations and their medicinal purpose. *Arnica montana,* for example, which, as its name suggests, grows in the mountainous regions of Europe and North America, is a specific remedy for the pain of fractures, sprains, muscle cramps, or overexertion.) Botanical medicine developed two strong branches through concentration on native growth as medicine. The exhaustive knowledge of regional medications merged with the developing techniques of "surgery" to form the ethnomedicine that remains, as noted, the dominant health care system in many pockets of the world. The other branch of pharmaceutical medicine, via returning travelers, missionaries, anthropologists, and scientific researchers, became integrated into orthodox "cosmopolitan" medicine. Experimentation around the world over many generations, though enhancing the knowledge of local medicines, confirmed hundreds of general and universal curatives that could be used in healing irrespective of time, place, or cultural beliefs.

Healing in a Hurry at Home

There remains, of course, a third theme of the folk tradition: "lay medicine," or "domestic medicine," as it was called in the nineteenth century, the broad and unorganized but persistent body of information that did *not* become integrated into either the formal indigenous medicines of Africa, Asia, and Europe or become part of the standard armamentarium of Western, scientific medicine. From this almost underground, folkloric, and intensely personal knowledge, we have inherited what some anthropologists call "rational folk medicine," a body of time-tested, improvisational, expedient substances and procedures that today form a storehouse of unsophisticated but helpful home remedies. They are passed on, not by shamans, priests, or recognized healers, nor by trained medicine men or doctors, but from generation to generation through daily contact within the families (or the latter-day versions of tribes) and communities, preserved by their repeated use in the empirical test of time.

Home remedies have distinct characteristics. They almost always involve common materials that are near at hand, plentiful, familiar, easy to use quickly in urgent situations, and generally known, in the case of plants and animal parts, to be edible and nonpoisonous. Another defining characteristic of a home remedy should probably be added: The recommended substance or procedure is something that has been used by an older member of the group. It is this "inherited" quality that demonstrates the apparently universal belief that the authority and presumed sagacity of the dispenser of cures is necessary and expected, whether the practitioner be a shaman, sorcerer, physician, psychotherapist—or grandmother. The range of such substances stretches from alfalfa to vinegar, from garlic to turpentine, from tree limbs to water, from baking soda to wheat bran. Many of them are used preventively to forestall disease and maintain good health, as well as curatively.

The line between domestic remedies and simple, good nutrition is sometimes blurred: For example, as useful as the lemon may be in dozens of distresses, it is also a chief ingredient of any good diet simply because of its broad contents of nutritive vitamins and minerals. As a result, it appears as a central ingredient in almost every cuisine in the world. Again, Pliny the Elder, in his *Natural History,* written almost two thousand years ago, observed the same overlap: "For a tiny sore a medicine is imported from the Red Sea, though genuine remedies form the daily dinner of even the poorest . . . but if remedies were sought in the kitchen garden . . . none of the arts would become cheaper than medicine."

Lemon Aid

The lemon, in fact, is a good example of the ideal home remedy. Certainly, though it cannot be grown in every climate, it is near at hand in most parts of the world, it is a common and familiar fruit in almost every culture, it is plentiful and relatively inexpensive even where it must be imported, and it is easy to use and is universally recognized as nontoxic. The juice of the lemon is, in fact, the most antiseptic liquid known to man, and more effective than rubbing alcohol or hydrogen peroxide.

Throughout the world the lemon is a central part of the domestic pharmacopoeia. The juice and rind are used not only for brushing the teeth and gums, where they kill bacteria, but, when mixed with saliva and the juice "chewed" slowly, help to remove plaque and tartar from the surface of the teeth. Likewise, the drinking of lemon juice (the juice of one lemon in 8 ounces of water, repeated up to 6 times a day) is a widespread practice all over the world as a general tonic for the body and to help calm the nerves. A variation of the morning lemon juice tonic is called the "morning drink" in India, where 2 tablespoons of honey and 2 tablespoons of lemon juice are mixed with only 1 ounce of water. (The leaves of the lemon, simmered for 20 minutes in 1½ cups of water, are used as a tea at night to help relax tension and aid sleep.)

The important active elements in lemon juice are vitamin C, calcium, potassium, a number of bioflavonoids, and of course citric acid. The lemon tree itself, usually a small, straggling tree from ten to fifteen feet high, was indigenous to Northern India and Burma. (The official botanical name, *limonun,* is derived from the Arabic *limun* or *limu,* which in turn may have come from the Sanskrit word *nimbuka.)* The trees reached Europe by way of Persia and were cultivated first in Greece, and then, in the second century, in Italy; lemons were established in the Western Hemisphere by Columbus, who had gathered seeds on one of his stops at the Canary Islands, and reintroduced them when he returned on his second trip to North America. Spanish explorers also carried lemon seeds to the New World in the sixteenth century, planting them in Mexico, Central America, and Florida. When the Franciscan fathers moved from Mexico to California two centuries later, they brought the seeds with them.

The distinguished naturalist Maud Grieve states flatly in her classic two-volume *A Modern Herbal,* that "it is probable that the lemon is the most valuable of all fruit for preserving health." Certainly, the lemon earned worldwide attention as a specific in the prevention and treatment of scurvy, the nutritional disorder caused by a deficiency of vitamin C (ascorbic acid). That disease, once common throughout Europe, especially where the local diet was lacking in fresh fruits or green vegetables and most of all among sailors who spent long periods at sea eating largely dried or salted foods, is characterized by extreme weakness, spongy gums, a tendency to develop hemorrhages under the skin and in the mucous membranes, and by mental depression and anemia. (So effective was lemon juice against these symptoms that for many years British ships were required by law to carry sufficient lemon or lime juice—the lime is a "cousin" species of the lemon—for every seaman to have an ounce daily after being ten days at sea. It was this practice, incidentally, that led to the popularization of the nickname "limey" to describe any English citizen.)

But the lemon and its juice and oil are not only antiscorbutic. Lemon juice is an effective diuretic, promoting the flow of urine, and an equally good diaphoretic, causing an increase in perspiration. These qualities have made it a standard domestic remedy for treating acute rheumatism, colds, flu, uric crystals, and even as a substitute for quinine (or synthetic drug) in treating malarial conditions. And, as I mentioned, the well-known astringent quality of the lemon has made it a universal home remedy as a gargle for sore throats and as a lotion in the event of sunburn. Many people believe that lemon juice is the best cure for severe, obstinate hiccoughs, and a gargle of lemon juice and warm water, alternated every hour with a gargle of warm, black leaf (nonherbal) tea is a remarkably effective treatment for intractable laryngitis. Surprisingly, considering the lemon's astringency, it has a long folk history as a cleansing eyewash: One drop (!) of fresh lemon juice in one eyecup (or one ounce) of warm water will clean and soothe eyes that have been exposed to dust or long hours under harsh lights. It is even claimed that the custom of using a slice of lemon when eating fish was not for flavoring or to "cut the taste" of the fish, but rather because people believed so strongly in the lemon's remedial power that they thought if a fish bone were unknowingly swallowed during the meal, the juice of the lemon would dissolve it.

In light of its enduring reputation as a healer, it seems likely that it was the lemon that inspired the text of Proverbs 8:19: "My fruit is better than gold, yea fine gold."

The Penicillin of Bees

In his fascinating and comprehensive book, *The Healing Hand,* the distinguished surgeon and historian of medicine Guido Majno tells of an experiment he designed to test the formula for a standard wound salve discovered in the so-called Smith Papyrus—an Egyptian text dating from between 2600 and 2200 B.C. The prescription called for a mixture of *ftt, mrht,* and *byt*—the words transliterated from hieroglyphic symbols: *ftt* signifying "lint, or some sort of vegetable fiber"; *mrht* meaning "grease"; and *byt,* or honey (the latter, Majno points out, was "by far the most popular Egyptian drug, being mentioned some five hundred times in nine hundred remedies).

In the contemporary experiments following a single reference in the Egyptian text suggesting a ratio of 1/3 to 2/3, Majno and his colleagues prepared a mixture of 1/3 honey to 2/3 fat, using either beef fat or butter. He writes: "It turned out that 1/3 honey is just right; more makes the paste too sticky. Despite the pleasant consistency, I thought at first that this would be dreadful stuff to put on an open wound. I visualized swarms of flies feeding on the honey, swarms of bacteria feeding on the sugar, and tissue reactions caused by the grease. When fatty substances are injected into the tissues they produce a persistent lump called a fat granuloma . . . to give the mixture the roughest possible test, we made it up with butter . . . which contains many bacteria of its own, including a group of coliform bacteria. Result: The bacteria initially present tended to disappear, and if pathogenic bacteria were added, like *Escherichia coli* or *Staphylococcus aureus,* they were killed just as fast." Majno's experiment confirmed what many other modern scientists have discovered: Honey is virtually harmless to tissues, it is aseptic, antiseptic, and antibiotic. Its powerful disinfectant quality stems from its hygroscopic action; that is, it draws moisture out of germs of all varieties, and germs, just as human beings, cannot survive without water. Experiments similar to Majno's, involving such deadly bacteria of the typhoid-colon group as *B. dysentariae, B. typhosus, B. paratyphosus A, B. paratyphosus B, B. proteus vulgaris,* and *B. coli communis,* resulted in *all* the bacteria being killed within ten hours to four days. Clearly, the Egyptians, Assyrians, Chinese, Greeks, and ancient Romans who employed honey both for wounds and the treatment of diseases of the liver, spleen, and digestive system, had discovered that the wild bee (since apiculture was not practiced in most of those societies) was producing from the nectar of flowers one of the most powerful and useful of natural drugs.

Honey contains, in varying degrees (depending on the soil in which the plants grew from which the bees extracted the nectar), iron, copper, manganese, silica, chlorine, calcium, potassium, sodium, phosphorus, aluminum, and magnesium, and a broad range of vitamins: B_1 (thiamine), B_2 (riboflavin), C (ascorbic acid), pantothenic acid, pyridoxine, and nicotinic acid. All these ingredients are nutritive, of course, and make honey valuable, and since honey nectar is predigested by the manufacturing bee, it is not only edible but is among the most digestible of foods. It has been used as a vehicle for mixing herbal preparations for internal consumption for probably fifteen thousand years, and the popularization of honey and vinegar as a "health-giving tonic" by the Vermont folk doctor D. C. Jarvis in the 1950s was anticipated seventeen centuries ago by the Spanish-born, Egyptian-educated physician Maimonides, who prescribed the same mixture, which he called "oxymel," to open up obstructions in the liver and spleen to stimulate the flow of urine and to help the intestines to evacuate excessive bile. Taken internally, or as an additive to herbal teas, honey has been used over the years to control muscle cramps, for athletic nutrition, to help produce sleep, as a trusted cough remedy, and in infant feeding.

The variety of uses to which honey may be put—in all these cases we are speaking of the pure, undiluted honey just as it comes from the hive and readily available from the nearest apiary or food store—makes it clearly one of nature's best self-administered remedies. But after all, as Majno has pointed out in marveling at the bee's ability to develop bactericidal nectar, "they have had 400 million years to work it out."

The Healer on the Windowsill

For thousands of years the *Aloe vera* plant, a member of the lily family, could not claim to be common and familiar anywhere but in Africa, the Mediterranean countries, or on certain West Indian islands. In eastern and southern Africa particularly, it was well known in ancient times, and it was even said the plant was used to prepare the body of Jesus for entombment. Throughout the Old World the aloe had religious significance not just for Christians: The Mohammedans considered it a holy plant; the Moslem who had made a pilgrimage to Mecca was entitled to hang the aloe over his doorway, and even the Jews of Cairo adopted the practice of hanging it up to protect the household from malign influences.

In the past twenty years, however, the remarkable medicinal properties of the *Aloe vera* have been rediscovered and analyzed, and though the plant is indigenous to tropical climates, it has been successfully naturalized as a houseplant even in colder areas; and for ease of maintenance it is virtually unmatchable. For one thing, it has, proportionately, one of the smallest root systems of any known plant, having developed over the centuries in a way that would permit its survival in an extremely dry climate where there may be no soil moisture for long periods of time. So unlike most plants, in which the leaves function to gather and transfer energy to the stem and root system, the lifeblood of the aloe is concentrated in the leaves, which, more than any other succulent, store an amazing amount of nutritives and moisture. Within those leaves are no less than eighteen amino acids, vitamins B_1, B_2, B_6, C, choline, niacinamide, and even the inorganic ingredients calcium, potassium, and chlorine. But above all, the leaves contain an assortment of anthraquinone glycosides, which are known collectively as "aloin."

Even though the *Aloe vera* has been approved by the Food and Drug Administration as a safe food additive, and the history of the plant's use internally is well documented, by all odds its best-known application is as an external ointment for tooth and gum pain, abrasions, burns, cuts, windburn, chafing, sunburn, insect bites, eczema, athlete's foot, fever blisters, poison ivy, poison oak, and the pain associated with joints and sore muscles.

The clear mucilaginous fluid obtained by cutting across and squeezing the spiky leaf of the aloe has remarkable effects: It anesthetizes the tissue in the area in which it is applied, it reduces bleeding time, reduces the heat or fever of sores, it is anti-inflammatory, it stops itching, and even breaks down and "digests" dead tissue (including pus) through the action of its proteolytic enzymes. At the same time, the aloe enhances normal cell proliferation, known as "epithelization," and thereby hastens the regenerative phase of the healing process. All this it does safely as an edible tropical fruit, in high concentration, and in direct contact with tissue, as opposed to synthetic drugs which might achieve the same range of benefits but, because of possible side effects, must be used only in limited doses and over a relatively long period of time.

In recent years the *Aloe vera* has been tested successfully, too, in the treatment of X-ray and other radiation burns, and in both the Soviet Union and the United States research is being done on the intravenous injection of the fluid of the plant as a treatment for tissue damaged by cobalt radiation (used in the nuclear treatment of cancer). Likewise, the gel is being tested for immediate application after surgery in an attempt to confirm the anecdotal evidence that its use will cause the incision to heal more rapidly and leave less of a scar.

There is no reason why this broad-spectrum, natural healer cannot become one of the basic domestic medicines in every household. The *Aloe vera* requires only modest amounts of light, very little water (during the winter it can go for several months without being watered), and in the summer, the small shoots which appear next to the mother plant can be removed and potted to form new plants. So enduring is this descendant of the lily that if a leaf of the *Aloe vera* is separated from the parent plant, it may be laid in the sun for several weeks without becoming entirely shriveled; and even when considerably dried by long exposure to heat, it will, if plunged into water, become plump, fresh, and useful within a few hours.

One can imagine no better use of a philanthropic grant than to put such a versatile and durable healing plant on every windowsill in the country.

Dangerous Magic

In a short story Isak Dinesen, the Danish writer who spent much of her life in the tribal villages of Africa, has one of her characters say, "Now cowdung is not actually a bad remedy for burns, since it coagulates quickly and will keep the air out." Indeed, the custom of using animal feces as a poultice for wounds and burns is one of the oldest emergency folk techniques in every recorded society. Like mud, it has been a ubiquitous and familiar substance wherever human beings have settled, and it is not hard to see why combinations of animal waste, dirt, sand, or leaves were grasped desperately to create improvised dressings for frightening wounds or burns. It has apparently always been clear that damaged flesh needs to be protected, either to prevent further chafing and abrasion or to protect it from air while the tissues try to mend themselves. One can imagine an isolated and severe enough occurrence even in modern times when anything available would seem to offer itself for this protection, even animal feces. But the fact is that this is one of the inherited medical traditions that should be avoided. We now know that in most places in the world, despite the assumption that the environment is sanitary and benign, the feces of animals are likely hosts for a broad range of infectious invasions (tetanus poisoning being the most probable) whose threat to life and health is far greater than the risks of leaving a burn uncovered.

Obviously, not all the folk traditions that have survived are appropriate or helpful now. The plants and foods and other substances that have worked in the past have clearly done so through chemical or biochemical means: They are effective not simply because they are convenient and "natural" but because, as we have seen in the case of lemons, honey, and *Aloe vera,* they are rich in strong chemicals science has defined as medicinal. By that same token, they contain chemical substances that either through overdosage or misapplication not only fail to heal, but are harmful. Despite the fact that most folk remedies have endured for centuries without evidence of harmful effects, and are especially noted for *not* causing uncomfortable or deleterious side effects, many should never be used, particularly by those who are neither skilled herbalists, physicians, or other well-trained practitioners.

The dangers are of three kinds: first, in the case of herbs or foods, the possibility of actual poisoning; second, as in the instance of animal feces used as a poultice, the risk of exposing a person to a secondary damage while treating a primary complaint; third, a combination of both possibilities. There has been a good deal of speculation that the painter Vincent van Gogh, who suffered from epilepsy, was continually under the effects of *Digitalis purpurea* (purple foxglove) in the latter part of his life— and the collateral symptoms it sometimes creates: xanthopsia (yellow vision), delirium, and restlessness—and that his affinity for the color yellow may have been caused or perpetuated by his medical treatment. (The possibility of toxicity in the use of digitalis also demonstrates the risks that attend certain substances, whether they are used in their "scientific" formulations or in the "natural" state. Withal that digitalis *may* be toxic, it is a prime example of an important and beneficial modern drug, the use of which derived directly from folk medicine.)

Those interested in using natural plants as remedies should also be alert to the fact that some plants may be good to eat or use medicinally at one time of the year and yet be poisonous at another time—poison ivy, chokecherries, and pokeweed, for example. These and other possibilities of internal poisoning or disturbing effects such as allergies, dermatitis, or mechanical injury due to scratching by prickles or thorns, are found throughout the botanical world and demand caution and knowledge. The following plants are known to be toxic in one way or another, and those interested in using plants for healing are urged to learn how to identify them, so they may be avoided:

apple-of-Peru	false hellebore	poison hemlock
baneberry	ground cherry	poison ivy and oak
beech	holly	pokeweed
black cherry	horse nettle	prickly poppy
black locust	hydrangea	rattlebox
black snakeroot	jack-in-the-pulpit	rayless goldenrod
bloodroot	jequirity pea	rhododendron
blue cohosh	jimsonweed	rock poppy
buckeye	Kentucky coffee tree	spurge
buckthorn	larkspur	spurge nettle
burning bush	lobelia	star-of-Bethlehem
buttercup	manchineel	stinging nettle
castor bean	May apple	strawberry bush
chinaberry	mescal bean	Virginia creeper
coontie	Mexican prickly poppy	water hemlock
corn cockle	mistletoe	white snakeroot
coyotillo	monkshood	wild balsam apple
cycads	moonseed	wild parsnip
dicentra	mountain laurel	yellow jasmine
dogbane	mulberry	yellow nightshade
elderberry	nightshade	yew
elephant's ear	oak (acorns)	

Likewise, though many herbalists and physicians disagree with the findings, and the subject is still being debated, the Food and Drug Administration has listed a number of herbs as "unsafe," so that those interested in using them should be aware that in certain dosages they may be toxic:

arnica	morning glory
belladonna	pennyroyal
bittersweet twigs	periwinkle
broom top	rue
calamus root	spindle tree
heliotrope	tonka bean
henbane	wahoo bark

jalap root   wormwood
lily-of-the-valley   yohimbé
mandrake

In the latter list belladonna is a good example of a plant that can be useful when the dosage is carefully monitored, as anyone can testify who has had a few drops of the extracted liquid inserted into the eyes in order to facilitate examination or for treatment of problems. Similarly, although pennyroyal and rue are doubtless on the FDA list because they may be dangerous when taken internally by a pregnant woman (who should also avoid ginger, tansy, rosemary, and black cohosh), they have a number of beneficial uses when used by others: Fresh, bruised rue leaves, for instance, can be applied directly to allay the pains of sciatica or headaches, and pennyroyal (a member of the mint family), is widely used as a tea in the treatment of flatulence, nausea, and stomach spasms.

For most of us, a number of commonsense cautions should be generally observed:

*Do not use unidentified herbs or plants.

*Do not use plants known to be narcotic.

*Use moderation when taking herbal preparations. Even in the case of unquestionably harmless substances, the doctrine of "more is better" is foolish. (After all, fatalities have been recorded from the extreme consumption of foods as innocuous as carrot juice or brown rice!)

*Do not take a large number of different herbs or plants at one time, or combinations of them. Quite apart from the distress that may be caused by the unknown effects of the mixture of these chemicals, the possible beneficial effects may be canceled out by the uninformed mixing of ingredients.

*As in the case of synthetic compounds, if a disturbing reaction develops after use of an herb or plant, such use should be discontinued, and the allergic reaction should be discussed with a trained medical practitioner.

*If a condition persists after ingesting a folk remedy—even if no negative response occurs—one should see a physician immediately. Folk remedies, like manufactured drugs, do not work uniformly for all people in all places and are not appropriate for every accident or illness. No matter how committed one may be to the use of "natural medicines," no condition should be allowed to go on without referral to a well-trained practitioner.

As for the folkloric traditions that may be relatively harmless in themselves but that might expose a patient to other, secondary risks, a comparable range of cautions should be observed:

*Never wrap a child who has a fever, but rather uncover him or her completely.

*Never put alcohol, tincture of iodine, lemon juice, or Merthiolate directly into a wound. Use soap and water.

*In addition to avoiding the use of feces on a burn or wound, never put grease, fat, hides, or coffee on such areas.

*Never rub or massage a broken limb or a limb that *may* be broken.

*Avoid castor oil or senna leaf as purgatives.

*Never use magnesium carbonate, milk of magnesia, or epsom salts as purges when there is pain in the belly.

*Never use dirt, kerosene, lime, lemon, or coffee to stop bleeding.

*Never give anything by mouth to a person who is unconscious.

*It is better to have no bandage at all than one that is dirty or wet.

New Healing in Old Prescriptions

The foregoing stand as really quite ordinary cautions in the use of any medication, and certainly do not form an argument against using natural substances and traditional first aid either in place of, or as adjuncts to, conventional treatments. As noted in Chap. 4, even more elaborate warnings are commonplace in the prescription of processed drugs and compounds. The human body is almost always involved in a dynamic biochemical process, and despite its remarkable inherent powers—including healing powers—it is vulnerable to reactions to substances and procedures introduced into that process.

Given that vulnerability, we might well ask why we use *any* materials or techniques to treat ourselves. If human nature is so mighty, why not simply let it take its course? The answer, of course, is that all medications are at least in part addressed to facilitating that natural healing ability. Synthetic or manufactured drugs for wounds and infection, for disease and disability, as well as the traditional treatments of our ancestors, are primarily intended to relieve the most painful and distressing immediate symptoms that disturb us and threaten our lives. The eventual achievement of healing, on the other hand, is accomplished by our own internal and external processes over a period of time *after* the initial treatment. No culture or society has developed without this principle at work; whatever explanation may have been consensual about the cause of accidents or illness, history records the universal human instinct to attempt to relieve pain, allay discomfort, restore mobility, and prolong life.

In light of this eternal drive to foster the healing process, it seems at best stubborn and at worst stupid to ignore the common, familiar, and traditional ways that our forebears used with success for so long. Many of those ways are characterized by simplicity and speedy effectiveness and are readily applicable by the lay person as well as the physician. The honey and myrrh of ancient Asia, the aloe and "arthritis root" of Africa, the acupressure points of China, the sweat baths of Native Americans, the tropical fruit juices of Central and South America, the slices of apples, onions, lemons, potatoes, and countless other foodstuffs of virtually every culture on the planet—the unique properties of all of these need only to be understood and respected in order to be restored to a medicine that aspires to completeness as well as to effectiveness and safety.

In our own age there are perhaps other and subtler reasons why the natural medicines of the ancients deserve attention and inclusion in professional medical institutions as well as domestic life. For one thing, urban populations all over the world are becoming increasingly polyglot communities, with new opportunities for the cross-fertilization of differing cultural traditions and the organized sharing of huge stores of rational folk medical practices. At the same time that large cities are changing in their characteristics, there are throughout the world enduring rural cultures, still intimately involved with the "old ways" and at the same time far removed from the facilities and the personnel of modern scientific medicine, which can affect them only intermittently. (The current attempt in China to integrate the herbal traditions, acupuncture, and moxibustion of the ancient times with modern Western medicine through the training of the "barefoot doctors" is an effort in the direction of this integration.) And, finally, the old traditions of self-curing in many cultures provide a rich stock of knowledge and skills that speak to the new movement throughout the world to promote self-care and mutual aid in small groups and communities that are attempting to regain control over the fundamental elements of their lives, such as energy sources, land use, the growing of nutritious foods, and the education of their children. For those who believe that in the past lie the seeds of restoration and balance in a world gone wrong through bigness and depersonalization, surely no part of a potential "whole medicine" could be richer than the intelligent use of the common ingredients of the environment in treating the ill and the wounded. No form of medical care could be more consistent with the principles of self-reliance and autonomy than the folk traditions that preceded industrialization and sophistication.

We need not, indeed should not, abandon the gains and the strivings of scientific medicine in order to share in the values of the folk tradition. We need only recognize that both may be valid at different times and for different purposes, and that there are more times than we are willing to admit when both can work together toward the goal of healing, which, as Richard Grossinger has written, "does not exist by permission of names; it exists in fact. Medicine thrusts into nature as it is, with all the local roughness and bias of things. Appropriate treatments are discovered in all cultures, as people are born, inhabit this world, and die."

PART II

NATURAL FIRST AID

Introduction

The tradition of first aid is as old as fire. The upright, mobile human being has always recognized that movement and activity involve risk. Whether the threat be wild animals, perilous terrain, or the winds and demons thought to be the source of illness and accidents, men and women have eternally needed to treat themselves with field expedients far from the shamans, the medicine men, or the physicians to whom they looked for expert treatment.

Nothing has been more fascinating in the evolution of human consciousness than the emergence of ingenuity and improvisation. The capacity to make any material at hand serve the purpose of survival—the limb of a nearby tree used in Colonial times to revive an unconscious man by suspending him upside down, later as a makeshift splint for a skier with a broken leg; the human mouth used in one instance to suck out poisonous venom and in another to breathe life into a drowning friend. Human imagination and invention have come out through the centuries, flowered most dramatically in crisis, each generation passing on to the next a storehouse of tricks and devices, procedures and stopgaps, manipulations and touches that, taken together, form an entire subspecialty within medicine.

But because first aid is influenced by medical theory, adapted for the accidental situation, it has been as culture-bound as formal medicine itself. The practice of first aid, therefore, has come to be limited to maneuvers derived from orthodox treatment in doctors' offices and hospitals. Such a system revises itself only as new things are learned in laboratory research. Thus, a mother in 1948 rushed for the butter when boiling soup spilled on her child's arm, while today that child, now a mother herself, rushes for ice, since burn treatment research has now confirmed that ice is more efficient than emollients in inhibiting the severity of tissue damage. Similarly, the boy who learned "artificial respiration" at summer camp in the 1930s now teaches his own children "cardiopulmonary resuscitation" (mouth-to-mouth breathing), and teaches the "Heimlich hug" for a choking emergency instead of a sharp slap between the shoulder blades. Such new approaches form the progressive evolution of first aid through *one* system—conventional Western medicine.

The other medical systems about which you have read in Part I of this book also contain an evolved body of knowledge and skills that may be used expediently for emergencies and other daily occurrences that call

143

for attention. Some are unchanged from the original form in which they were first used thousands of years ago; some are latter-day developments arising from the ongoing practice of ancient therapies in many parts of the world. Because so many of these unorthodox medical practices are aspects of cultural, philosophical, and religious beliefs regarding the need and virtue of autonomy and self-responsibility, the first aid component of their therapies is particularly suited to self-treatment of symptoms, and these practices are easy to learn and apply in mundane situations. From the skinned knees of children to persistent tooth and gum pain, the common distresses of daily life are universal, and the other medicines offer a particularly rich array of techniques that can readily be employed by anyone to relieve pain and anxiety and in many instances restore complete mobility.

Readers are urged to read the introductory material that precedes the specific procedures described. A familiarity with the limitations and contraindications for "natural" medical techniques is as important as recognizing the possibility of negative reactions to synthetic drugs, and if any distressing responses occur, of course, the "natural" procedure should be stopped at once.

As with the familiar first aid techniques of conventional Western medicine, the procedures described in the following pages are intended for emergency use, and whenever possible should be accompanied, or quickly followed, by consultation with a physician or other qualified medical practitioner.

Notes on Using Herbs

The fact that many plants and herbs are recommended in this book as being effective for the relief of a wide range of symptoms does not imply a blanket assumption that any "natural" substance is, by definition, safe for medical use. The very qualities in herbs that *do* make them effective are chemical in nature, and it is well established that some of those chemical components in excessive dosages are not only not helpful, but even dangerous.

You will not find, therefore, any of the following plants prescribed for internal use in this book, and you are strongly urged not to use them even though you have heard about them from friends or family members:

apple-of-Peru	dogbane	monkshood
arnica	elderberry	moonseed
baneberry	elephant's ear	morning glory
beech	false hellebore	mountain laurel
belladonna	ground cherry	mulberry
bittersweet twigs	heliotrope	mushrooms
black cherry	henbane	nightshade
black locust	holly	oak (acorns)
black snakeroot	horse nettle	pennyroyal
bloodroot	hydrangea	periwinkle
blue cohosh	jack-in-the-pulpit	poison hemlock
broom top	jalap root	poison ivy and oak
buckeye	jequirity pea	pokeweed
buckthorn	jimsonweed	prickly poppy
burning bush	Kentucky coffee tree	rattlebox
buttercup	larkspur	rayless goldenrod
calamus root	lily-of-the-valley	rhododendron
castor bean	lobelia	rock poppy
chinaberry	mandrake	rue
coontie	manchineel	spindle tree
corn cockle	May apple	spurge
coyotillo	mescal bean	spurge nettle
cycads	Mexican prickly poppy	star-of-Bethlehem
dicentra	mistletoe	stinging nettle

strawberry bush   white snakeroot   yellow jasmine
tonka bean   wild balsam apple   yellow nightshade
Virginia creeper   wild parsnip   yew
wahoo bark   wormwood   yohimbé
water hemlock

Measuring Herbs

The simplest way to measure dried herbs is to determine their ounce weight on a pan balance scale, which can be bought at some drugstores or by mail from a scientific supply house. Gram scales are also available, usually for under fifty dollars, and good quality kitchen scales may be purchased for less than twenty dollars. The following tables will be helpful in computing the amounts of herbs you use:

Weights and Measures

1 pound = 453 grams
1 ounce = 28.3 grams
16 ounces (dry) = 1 pound
1 quart = 2 pints
1 pint = 2 cups
1 cup = 16 ounces (fluid)
1 teaspoon = 60 drops
1 tablespoon = 3 teaspoons
1 fluid ounce = 2 tablespoons
1 cup = 16 tablespoons

Capsules and Powders

15.4 grains = 1 gram
1 gram = 1000 milligrams (mg)

Contents of 1 "00" capsule = about 650 mg = 10 grains
Contents of 1 "0" capsule = about 500 mg = 8 grains
2 gelatin capsules = 1 teaspoon of the tincture
2 tablespoons tincture = 1½ cup of tea

1 teaspoon of powder will fill about 2 "00" capsules
1 ounce of powdered herbs will therefore fill 40
   to 50 "00" capsules, or 50 to 70 "0" capsules,
   depending on the type of herb, the fineness of
   powder, and the tightness of packing.

The Qualities of Herbs

Alterative: Nonspecific action which improves the general functioning of body parts and, when taken over a long period of time, favorably alters the course of the ailment.

Anodyne: Allays pain.

Anthelmintic: Eliminates or destroys intestinal worms.

Antiseptic: Destroys and/or checks growth of harmful bacteria.

Antispasmodic: Relieves or stops spasms, convulsions, or cramps.

Aperient: Acts as a gentle, nonpurging laxative.

Carminative: Expels gas from alimentary canal.

Chologogue: Increases the flow of bile.

Coagulant: Promotes blood clotting.

Demulcent: Soothes and protects irritated tissues, particularly mucous membranes.

Deobstructant: Opens passages of the body.

Diaphoretic: Promotes involuntary perspiration.

Diuretic: Increases secretion and flow of urine.

Emetic: Induces vomiting.

Emmenagogue: Promotes menstruation.

Emollient: Softens and soothes inflamed tissues.

Expectorant: Promotes discharge of mucus.

Febrifuge: Reduces and abates fever.

Hemostatic: Stops bleeding.

Hepatic: Affects the liver.

Laxative: A mild purgative.

Nervine: Soothes the nerves.

Parturient: Helps to induce childbirth.

Pectoral: Clears and relieves respiratory tract.

Purgative: Causes the thorough emptying of the bowels.

Refrigerant: Reduces body heat.

Rubefacient: Increases circulation and produces slight reddening of the skin.

Sedative: Relieves tension, soothes nerves.

Stimulant: Produces temporary quickening of a vital process.

Stomachic: Promotes gastric digestion.

Tonic: Invigorates and strengthens entire body.

Vermifuge: Expels worms.

Vulnerary: Heals wounds.

How to Make Herbal Preparations

Always use ceramic, glass, or enamel containers. Do not use metal, especially aluminum.

Infusion

Pour 2 cups boiling water over 1 ounce (about 1 tablespoon) dried herbs or 1 loose handful of fresh herbs. Steep at least 10 minutes. This is often called a "standard brew." A little pure honey may be added. The usual dose is a small cupful 3 or 4 times a day.

Decoction

Soak 1 ounce dried herb, root, seeds, or bark in 2 cups cold water for several hours; bring to a boil and simmer for 1/4 hour. Cool. Honey may be used. The usual dose is 1/2 cup before meals.

Fomentation

Dip clean cloth in unsweetened infusion or decoction. Wring out excess and apply externally.

Embrocation

Dilute a decoction in a gallon of water and use warm for soaks.

Tincture

Pour 1 pint of pure alcohol or brandy over 2 ounces of dried herbs or a large handful of fresh herbs in a glass jar with a cap. Close the jar tightly and turn upside down. Shake the jar once or twice a day for a week. Strain and return liquid to the jar. Tinctures keep up to 6 months. The usual dose is 1 tablespoon to a wineglass of water, once or twice a day.

Standard Brew Concentrate for Cough Syrup

Make an infusion of 8 ounces of herbs to 12 ounces of water. Steep 20 minutes. Add equal amount pure honey. The usual dose is 2 teaspoons in 1/2 glass warm water, 2 or 3 times daily.

Poultice

For external use chop fresh or dried herbs, moisten with apple cider vinegar, and mix with whole wheat flour or cooked barley as binder. Spread on a moist, hot cloth. Place over lightly oiled skin. A heating pad (low setting) may be placed on top, or cover poultice with a piece of plastic to retain the heat.

Salve

Cover herbs with water; bring to a boil and simmer for 30 minutes. Strain and add an equal amount of olive or safflower oil. Simmer until only the oil is left. Add enough beeswax to achieve salve consistency. Pour while hot into a glass jar. It will keep up to one year.

Notes on Using Acupressure Points

Locating Points

The measurements of distances between points and in relation to parts of the body are given in "finger widths." This is meant to indicate the finger widths of patients. For example, to locate the points for menstrual cramps (see page 171), the patient (or you, if you are treating yourself) should lay the first four fingers of one hand laterally across the opposite ankle, with the little finger crossing the peak of the shinbone. As the illustration indicates, the points are then located behind the back edge of the long muscle in your leg. (The specific point is often identifiable because it is more sensitive to touch than the surrounding area.)

Pressing Technique

The Chinese practice of *Tui-Na* (literally, "pushing, grabbing") consists of 16 different methods for manipulating the points on the meridians to help restore the balance of *ch'i:* pushing, patting, vibrating, twisting, brushing, kneading, pounding, rolling, bending, pressing, rubbing, "ironing," picking, plucking, digging, and pointing. Of all these refinements, the basic technique recommended in this book is simple pressure and rotation. The rule as to depth of pressure is "beyond pleasure, but short of pain." For the procedures covered in this book, pressure of the thumb, index finger, or middle finger is usually indicated, meaning the padded tip of those fingers, though in several instances instructions call for using the nail of the finger. Pressure is applied while rotating the finger 2 to 3 cycles per second.

Important Notes

Your hands should be warm when you use acupressure on yourself or others. Wash your hands in warm water before proceeding, and/or rub them briskly together. When applying the pressure, try to be as relaxed as possible, breathing in slowly while pressing the point and slowly breathing out as pressure is released.

Do not use acupressure, or recommend it for others, in the following instances:

1. Before or after eating a heavy meal.
2. Before or after bathing in hot water.
3. During pregnancy, especially after the third month.
4. Within four hours after taking any drugs, alcohol, or medications that affect perception or equilibrium.
5. If the pressure point falls on an open wound or other vulnerable place on the skin.

The duration of acupressure procedures are specified in the text. Procedures may be repeated as necessary, but generally acupressure should not be used for more than one hour at any one time. Where points occur bilaterally on the body, both points should be pressed. (See illustration below for nausea, for example.)

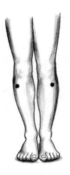

Notes on Using Yogic Therapy

The recommendations for the appropriate ways to use Yogic therapy are bound up with the original religious practice of Yogic tradition. Modern teachers realize that a different cultural environment makes it impossible to follow the old hard-and-fast rules however.

Nevertheless, except for lavages and those procedures used for emergency purposes, the Yogic meditations and breathing exercises are most helpful when employed in the following circumstances:

*Practice in the early morning and after sunset.
*For most people, sessions should be between 15 and 30 minutes long.
*The best seasons in which to begin are spring and autumn, when the weather is mild.
*Practice in a clean, airy place, as free from distracting noise as possible. Try to use the same spot regularly.
*Breathe through the nose only.
*Keep your eyes closed throughout your exercises, and remain sensitive to the sound and quality of your breath.
*Stop any exercise immediately if you experience dizziness, pressure or ringing in the ears, or if rhythmic breathing becomes strained.

Notes on Using Homeopathic Preparations

Of the over two thousand animal, vegetable, and mineral substances used in formal homeopathic treatment, this book deals with only twenty-eight remedies. They are among those used most often for the minor ailments and injuries covered here.

These twenty-eight remedies are contained in a kit prepared by one of the leading homeopathic pharmaceutical houses, Luyties Pharmacal Company in St. Louis, Missouri, and is distributed by the National Center for Homeopathy, 7297-H Lee Highway, Falls Church, Virginia 22044, for a cost of about thirty dollars. Similar kits of assorted remedies for home use are available from Homeopathic Educational Services, 5916 Chabot Crest, Oakland, California 94618, and John A. Bornemann & Sons, Inc., 1208 Amosland Road, Norwood, Delaware County, Pennsylvania 19074. (Of course, individual remedies in tablet or liquid form may be purchased directly from one of the retail pharmacies which carry them; many health food stores are also beginning to stock at least a modest assortment of homeopathic medications.)

The remedies in the Home Remedy Kit are all 6x potency, which, you will recall, means that the original substance has been diluted and shaken in six stages of mixture with a water and alcohol compound (see Chap. 5). 6x is considered a "low potency," with higher potencies being used for chronic conditions, and such higher potencies should be dispensed only by physicians. But because 6x is low does not mean that it is "weak"; if the correct remedy is used, its action can be truly powerful.

Remembering that, unlike allopathic medications, the homeopathic remedies are not designed to "fight and destroy" pain or infection, but are intended to enhance your natural self-healing powers, the question arises as to how homeopathic pellets or tinctures can be listed as "specifics." It is true that in full-fledged homeopathic practice, medications are not generalized as being "for" conditions, but are prescribed only when the fullest possible *unique* profile of the ailing person is established by interview and examination. Homeopathy, it should be remembered, does not treat conditions, it ministers to people.

However, in the over two hundred years since Samuel Hahnemann first developed homeotherapeutics, a number of "basic" remedies have been found to be helpful in the relief of acute and localized symptoms. The general rules of homeopathy, however, should be observed:

*Observe the law of similars; that is, match the symptoms of the patient as closely as you can to the symptoms that were produced in healthy people when they were part of "proving" experiments. (The kit includes six pamphlets under the general title of *Family Self-Help Using Homeopathy* which will assist you, or you may use one of the homeopathic texts described in the Annotated Bibliography. Of these, one of the best is *Homeopathic Medicine at Home* by Dr. Maesimund Panos and Jane Heimlich. Dr. Panos also prepared the pamphlets in the Home Remedy Kit.)

*Give or take only one remedy at a time, and do not use any remedy unnecessarily, or in larger than recommended doses.

*If there is no relief within one hour, you have probably selected the incorrect remedy and need to reassess the ill or injured person. Discontinue the remedy as soon as you observe that improvement is well established.

*Homeopathic medications should be taken, as much as possible, with a "clean" mouth—free of food, tobacco, toothpaste, mouthwash, candy, or any other substance except plain water. The ideal time to take a remedy is in the morning before brushing the teeth or eating breakfast. For fifteen minutes before or after taking a remedy, put nothing in the mouth, and take the tablets directly under the tongue where they will dissolve quickly and be absorbed directly by the mucous membranes.

*Never transfer remedies from their original containers. Keep them away from heat, strong light, and pervasive odors such as menthol, mothballs, camphor, and perfume.

*Store all homeopathic remedies as securely as you would any other medications. Although they are nontoxic substances, even to infants, the household rule of assuring that children do not have access to drugs should be observed.

PROCEDURES
FOR
COMMON
COMPLAINTS

Abrasions and Burns

◆ For first-degree burns, immediately plunge the affected part into cold water and soak for at least 3 minutes. Do not use butter, margarine, or other grease or oils.

◆ The mucilaginous fluid in the leaf of the *Aloe vera* plant is an anodyne, a demulcent, and an emollient. Break a leaf from the plant, slit it open, and apply directly to burns and abrasions by squeezing the liquid onto the wound or by rubbing the slit leaf on the skin. The fluid is also effective for pimples, chapped or roughened areas, and sunburn.

◆ Apply grated raw potato or a poultice of bread soaked in hot milk.

◆ A grated raw onion, lightly salted, will be helpful. (Use only a freshly sliced onion, since the onion absorbs bacteria in the environment.)

◆ A few grains of sugar sprinkled on the tongue will relieve the distress of tongues burned with hot food or drink. Repeat as often as needed.

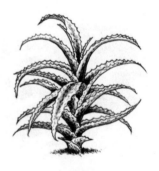

Aloe Vera

Homeopathy: Cantharis alleviates the pain of burns and scalds.

157

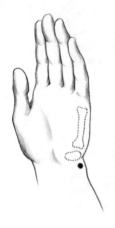

Anxiety Reactions, Acute

Acupressure Points: On the skin crease of the wrist on the ulnar side. Use *thumbnail* to press hard. **Apply pressure and rotate thumbnail for 2 to 3 minutes. Both** wrists.

Yogic Breathing: Breathe in slowly through the nose, filling the abdomen and lowering the diaphragm. After the abdomen is filled and expanded, complete the breath by continuing to inhale, filling the chest with air and raising it. Exhale *slowly* and completely from the upper chest, then from the abdomen. Repeat several times.
◆   Peppermint tea is helpful in calming the nerves. (One heaping teaspoon of leaves in 1 cup of boiling water. Drink freely.)
◆   A standard infusion of valerian, taken cold, is helpful. Drink no more than 2 cups per day.

Homeopathy: Aconite *(Aconitum napellus)* if anxiety is the effect of fright or shock. *Ignatia amara* is the "grief remedy" when there has been emotional upset and the patient sighs frequently.

Colds and Congestion

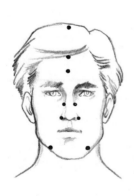

Acupressure Points I: Follow the sequence in the drawing: (1) on both sides of the nose as it begins to flare; (2) at the base of the nostril; (3) at the beginning of the flare of the lower jaw; (4) at the top center point of the skull, in the midline of the nose; (5) at the hairline (or four finger widths above the eyebrows), also in the midline of the nose; and (6) on the forehead in the midline. Press firmly and rotate with thumbs or fingers. Press the entire sequence for 3 to 5 minutes. Repeat as necessary.

Acupressure Points II: Over the back of the hand, between the bones of the thumb and index finger. Use the thumb to press firmly and rotate against the index fingers. Both hands. (Note: The point is also used for headache, acute pain, and toothache.)

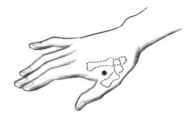

Acupressure Points III: At the space between the C-7 and T-1 spinal vertebrae. (The C-7 spinal process is the one that protrudes when the head and neck are bent forward slightly. The T-1 spinal process is immediately below it.) Use the tip of the index finger to press and massage for 2 minutes. Then, 2 inches to each side of the space between T-2 and T-3, press firmly and rotate the thumbs for 2 minutes.

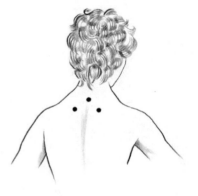

Yogic Therapy I: To clear slightly blocked nostrils, apply pressure with fingers, pushing up into the central portion of the armpit opposite the affected nostril. Release pressure after 3 seconds. Repeat as needed.

Yogic Therapy II: (Lavage) Mix 1/2 teaspoon salt, 1/8 teaspoon baking soda with 1 cup of hot water (test heat by touching wetted finger to the inside of the nostril). Bend your head forward and downward. Let your lower jaw be slack as you open your mouth. With your nose, slowly inhale a small amount of the mixture with your jaw and palate in this relaxed position. Continue to inhale the mixture to the back of the throat but without swallowing it. Spit out the water vigorously through your mouth. Repeat until cup is empty.

Home Remedies:
◆ Hot lemonade taken before bedtime induces perspiration and reduces congestion.

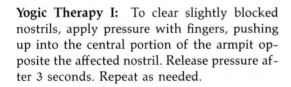

◆ Hot chicken soup relieves congestion, as does plain hot water.
◆ Hot, spicy foods with garlic, chilies, or cayenne pepper relieve congestion.
◆ Garlic tablets or capsules can be helpful in relieving respiratory infections.

Herbal Teas and Inhalants:
◆ Infusion of yarrow, rose hips, peppermint, or sage. Drink freely.
◆ Infusions of catnip or vervain relieve colds and fevers by inducing perspiration and calming.
◆ Ginger tea, made by steeping ½ ounce of the powdered root in one pint of boiling water for 15 minutes.
◆ Place a handful of peppermint or chamomile in a pot of boiling water; put a towel over the head and make a tent. Breathe in the vapors through the nose.
◆ 1 teaspoon salt in a glass of warm water as a gargle.

Homeopathy: *Allium cepa* for beginning colds with frequent sneezing and watery eyes. *Gelsemium sempervirens* if there are complaints of dullness, aching, and chills, the patient is not thirsty, and for "summer colds." *Phosphorus* for a chest cold; *Pulsatilla* for an advanced (ripe) cold with profuse yellowish discharge from the nose.

Colic

Herbal Teas: Warm chamomile or catnip tea, sweetened with honey. Infuse ¼ teaspoon chamomile to 1 cup boiling water. Steep 5 to 10 minutes. Up to 1 ounce (2 tablespoons) of warm mixture; repeat as needed.

Homeopathy: *Nux vomica,* or *Chamomilla* if attack is associated with exposure to cold weather.

Constipation

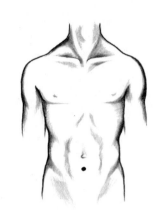

Acupressure Point: About 4 inches below the navel along the midline of the body. With patient supine, use thumb or palm to press hard, 1 to 3 minutes.

Home Remedies:
♦ Regular inclusion of whole grain and wheat bran in the diet helps to prevent constipation.
♦ Figs, prunes, pears, and rhubarb are all laxatives.
♦ Olive oil (1 teaspoon as a mild laxative).
♦ 5 to 10 drops of tincture of cascara sagrada (available at most pharmacies) taken in water, before meals.

Homeopathy: *Nux vomica* (especially if constipation alternates with diarrhea), or *Ignatia amara.*

Coughs

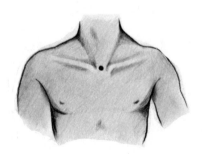

Acupressure Points: In the depression above the front notch of the collarbones, press index finger inward, then massage downward for 2 minutes.

Home Remedies: 1 teaspoon honey, or a mixture of honey and lemon juice.

Herbal Teas:
♦ Make an infusion of St.-John's-wort. Drink 3 or 4 cups daily.
♦ For spasmodic cough: an infusion of black cohosh.
♦ Make an infusion of horehound or horehound and comfrey. Drink 3 or 4 cups daily.

◆ To loosen bronchial secretions, use an infusion of elecampane (sweetened with honey).

Herbal Inhalants: Place a handful of eucalyptus leaves in a pot of boiling water. Put a towel over the head to make a tent. Breathe in the vapors through the nose.

Herbal Cough Medicine: Prepare horehound or coltsfoot, together or separately, in a standard brew concentrate (8 ounces of herbs, 12 ounces of water; infuse for 20 minutes). Add an equal amount of honey. Take 2 teaspoons in 1/2 glass of warm water, 3 or 4 times daily.

Homeopathy: *Belladonna* for a barking cough; *Hepar sulphuris calcareum* for a loose croupy, or choking cough; *Carbo vegetabilis* for a convulsive cough; *Bryonia* for a dry, hard, or gagging cough; *Spongia* for a dry croupy cough; for a wheezing cough, *Antimonium tartaricum.*

Diarrhea

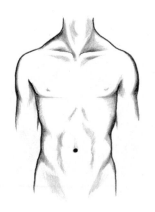

Acupressure Point: Right at the navel. Use palm or thumb to press and rotate gently, 1 to 3 minutes.

Herbal Teas:
◆ Infuse 1 teaspoon ginger root in 1 cup of boiling water. Drink 3 cups per day.
◆ Infuse 1 ounce peppermint, mullein, or yarrow in 2 cups of boiling water. Drink freely.
◆ Put 1 ounce powdered slippery elm into 1 quart of boiling water; simmer down the mixture to 1 pint. Dosage: 1 teaspoon every half hour, with honey if needed.

Home Remedy: 1 1/2 ounces of blackberry brandy, sipped slowly.

Homeopathy: *Bryonia,* if diarrhea alternates with constipation; after cold drinks or food in hot weather, use *Arsenicum album;* if associated with cold weather, *Ipecacuanha* or *Nux vomica;* if accompanied by sweating and weakness, *Veratrum album.*

Earache

Home Remedy: Boil 1 clove of garlic in ½ cup of water until soft (not mushy). Lay cool clove on the *outside* of the ear—do not insert in ear canal. Repeat daily for several days. Or, use one drop of warm, not hot, garlic oil in the ear, once a day.

Homeopathy: *Ferrum phosphoricum.*

Eye Problems

Herbal Eyewash: 1 ounce eyebright *(Euphrasia officinalis)* in 1 cup boiling water. After boiling, allow to cool, and use in eyecup. Repeat as needed. Or use 1 drop (!) of fresh lemon juice in 1 ounce of warm, not hot, water. Use an eyecup or small paper cup.

Eyestrain
Moisten cottonballs with witch hazel; place on eyelids for 10 to 15 minutes. (See "Palming" exercise, p. 186.)

Eye Swelling
◆ Herbal poultice: Place 1 or 2 bruised ivy leaves on the eyelid. Leave on for 15 minutes.
◆ Place freshly sliced cucumber on eyelids. Leave for 10 to 15 minutes.
◆ Place moistened tea bags of black tea (e.g.,

orange pekoe) on eyelids for 10 to 15 minutes.

Homeopathy: *Aconitum napellus* will relieve the pain in eye injuries.

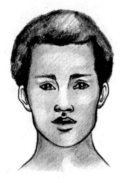

Fainting

Acupressure Points I: Just above the middle of the depression on the surface of the upper lip, one third down from the base of the nose, two thirds up from the top edge of the upper lip. Use thumbnail or index fingernail and press hard.

Acupressure Point II: At the upper one third of the sole of the foot, on a line between the second and third toes. Use the thumbnail to press hard. Both feet.

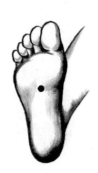

Homeopathy: *Spongia,* or, if it occurs on least exertion, *Veratrum album.* For sudden fear associated with restlessness, *Aconitum napellus.*

Flatulence

Herbal Teas:
◆ Infusions of catnip, chamomile, peppermint, bee balm (bergamot), fennel, anise seeds, dill, or sage.
◆ Ginger tea or an infusion of cloves.

Homeopathy: *Carbo vegetabilis* or *Nux vomica.*

Hay Fever

Herbal Tea: An infusion of red clover blossoms; drink 3 to 4 cups daily before expected contact, 6 to 8 cups daily if an attack occurs or during the height of the season.

Home Remedy: Progressive desensitization can be achieved by chewing 1 teaspoon daily of the cappings from *local* honey. Chew until only a bit of wax remains, and spit it out. Do this daily for 1 month prior to usual onset of hay fever. Also eat local, unprocessed honey.

Headache, Frontal

Acupressure Points: Follow the sequence in the drawing: (1) About 2 finger widths below the top center point of the skull, in the midline of the nose; (2) at the hairline (or 4 finger widths above the eyebrows), in the midline; (3) on the forehead, in the midline; and (4) between the eyebrows. Use middle finger to press firmly and rotate. Complete the entire sequence for 2 to 3 minutes. Repeat as necessary.

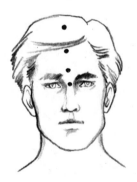

Headache, Migraine

Acupressure Point I: About 1 finger width above the peak of the eyebrow, vertical to the pupil.

Acupressure Point II: 1 inch from the side corner of the eye. Use middle finger to press and rotate firmly for 2 to 3 minutes.

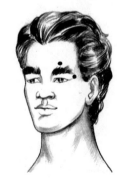

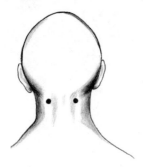

Headache, Occipital

Acupressure Point: Just below the lower edge of the skull, to the side of the depressions on both sides. Press and rotate for 2 to 3 minutes, both sides.

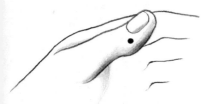

Headache, One-sided

Acupressure Point: Approximately ⅛ inch behind the corner of the thumbnail on the radial side of the thumb, on the same side as the headache. Use thumbnail to press and rotate for 2 to 3 minutes.

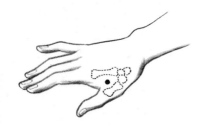

Headache, General

Acupressure Point: Over the dorsum of the hand, between the first and second metacarpal bones (the thumb and first finger). Use the thumb of the other hand to press firmly and rotate against the index finger. Both hands.

Homeopathy: If pain is bandlike around the entire head, *Gelsemium sempervirens*. If open air improves it, or it is dull and worse in the evening, *Allium cepa*.

Herbal Teas: Infusions of peppermint, chamomile, catnip, vervain, or feverfew are used.

Herbal Inhalants: Inhale the steam produced by placing a handful of peppermint or wintergreen in a pot of boiling water. Put a towel over the head to create a tent.

Poultice: Warmed cod liver oil on cotton flannel applied locally to the chest or the forehead.

Breathing and Relaxation:
◆ Headaches resulting from teeth clenching during sleep can be eliminated by the following practice: Clench teeth and let go 5 times, repeating the exercise 5 times daily.
◆ Many headaches can be relieved by the breathing and relaxation techniques described on pp. 183 and 186.

Mental Imagery: Combining the visualization of a white light that fills the head and replaces the headache together with breathing and complete body relaxation relieves headaches.

Hiccoughs

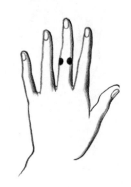

Acupressure Points I: On both sides of the second joint of the middle finger. Use the thumbnail to press hard. Both hands.

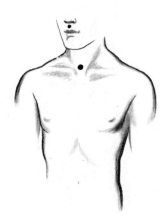

Acupressure Points II: Simultaneously, right on the front notch of the collarbones and at the point located between the nose and the top edge of the upper lip. Using both middle fingers, press firmly on these two points.

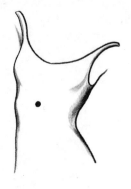

Acupressure Points III: About 4 fingers width below the sternum in line with the navel. Use middle finger to press firmly and rotate.

Hysteria

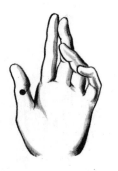

Acupressure Point: At the center of the bottom crease of the thumb. Use the thumbnail to press hard. Both thumbs.

Herbal Teas: Infusions of lavender or peppermint.

Indigestion

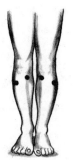

Acupressure Point I: Just below the knee, in the depression on the inner part of the leg. Use thumb to press and rotate firmly.

Acupressure Point II: 4 finger widths below the apex of the kneecap, 1 finger width to the side of the tibia (the large bone in front of the leg). Press firmly with the thumb or middle finger and rotate 2 to 4 minutes.

Herbal Teas: Infusion of one half sweet woodruff and one half St.-John's-wort. Chamomile, peppermint, vervain, and ginger teas are also useful for digestive distress.

Homeopathy: *Carbo vegetabilis,* especially if belching occurs; *Arsenicum album* if food poisoning is involved; *Nux vomica,* especially after overeating or in the event of a hangover.

Stomach Stretch (requires two persons): Stand back-to-back with both arms intertwined. One person slowly bends forward, bearing the weight of the patient over the length of his or her spine, lifting the patient gently off the floor in an outstretched position. Patient should be encouraged to be in as totally relaxed a position as possible. Hold for 1 minute. Repeat the lift 2 or 3 times if necessary.

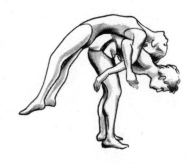

Insect Bites and Stings

Herbal Treatment: Crush a few plantain leaves, and apply the juice to the skin for relief of bites.

Home Remedies:
◆ Break a leaf from the *Aloe vera* plant, slit it open and apply directly by squeezing the liquid or rubbing the slit leaf on the skin for bites.
◆ Moisten 1/3 teaspoon of unseasoned meat tenderizer with one teaspoon of water, and apply.

Homeopathy: *Apis mellifica.* Externally, use either tincture of *Ledum, Arnica,* or *Hypericum.*

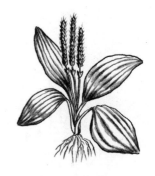

Plantain

Stings, Bee and Wasp

Home Remedies:
◆ Bicarbonate of Soda: Moisten bicarbonate of soda with water and apply as a paste to bee and wasp stings.
◆ Onion: A slice of peeled raw onion applied to bee and wasp stings draws out swelling and lessens pain.
◆ Fresh Lemon Juice or Vinegar: Apply directly to mosquito bites.

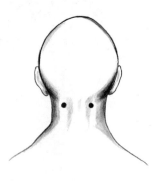

Insomnia

Acupressure Point I: Just below the lower edge of the skull, to the side of the depressions on both sides. Press firmly and rotate both points 2 to 3 minutes.

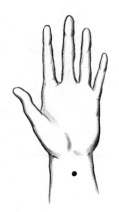

Acupressure Points II: Two fingers width down from the skin crease of the wrist, between the two large tendons. Both wrists.

Herbal Teas: Drink infusions of chamomile tea, or one half sweet woodruff and one half St.-John's-wort, or lemon balm, or vervain, all mild sedatives. Most herb stores carry a mixture, usually consisting of hops, skullcap, valerian, catnip, peppermint, chamomile, and mullein. One cup about one hour before retiring aids sleep.

Home Remedies:
◆ Warm milk contains high concentrations of the amino acid tryptophan, which appears to have sedative qualities.
◆ A teaspoon of honey acts as a mild sedative.

Homeopathy: *Arsenicum album* or *Belladonna* may be helpful.

Yogic Breathing and Total Body Relaxation: Abdominal breathing, coupled with clockwise or counterclockwise rubbing of the abdomen 81 times is recommended. (See instructions on p. 183.)

Laryngitis

Herbal Tea: An infusion of marshmallow used as a gargle and drunk as a tea, is useful.

Home Remedy: Alternate hourly a gargle of diluted fresh lemon juice (juice of 1/4 lemon to 5 ounces of warm water) and a gargle of black tea (e.g., orange pekoe). Continue over a two-day period.

Yogic Lavages: See p. 159 for instructions.

Menstrual Problems (cramps and edema)

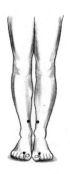

Acupressure Points I: 4 fingers width above the peak of the shinbone, on the long muscle. Rotate thumb or index finger firmly for 2 to 4 minutes for cramps.

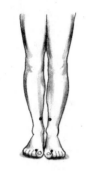

Acupressure Points II: On the depression between the big toe and the first toe. Rotate thumb or index finger firmly for 2 to 4 minutes for cramps.

Herbal Teas: Chamomile, strawberry or raspberry leaf, blue cohosh, catnip, horehound, lemon balm, squaw vine, comfrey root with peppermint, ginger, made into infusions. Drink 3 to 4 cups daily for cramps. Dandelion tea is diuretic.

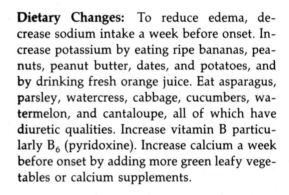

Dietary Changes: To reduce edema, decrease sodium intake a week before onset. Increase potassium by eating ripe bananas, peanuts, peanut butter, dates, and potatoes, and by drinking fresh orange juice. Eat asparagus, parsley, watercress, cabbage, cucumbers, watermelon, and cantaloupe, all of which have diuretic qualities. Increase vitamin B particularly B_6 (pyridoxine). Increase calcium a week before onset by adding more green leafy vegetables or calcium supplements.

Massage: A complete foot massage (no longer than 15 minutes) is helpful in relaxing tension throughout the body. (See p. 192 for instructions.)

The Cobra

Yogic Postures: "The cobra" and "the bow" are recommended. (See illustrations.)

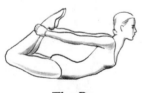

The Bow

Homeopathy: For excessive flow, *Arsenicum album;* for painful cramps, *Chamomilla or Aconitum napellus.*

Motion Sickness

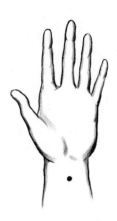

Acupressure Point: 2 finger widths below the skin crease of the wrist, between the two large tendons. Both wrists.

Herbal Treatment: Dry ginger in capsules or ginger tea are useful.

Homeopathy: *Hypericum* or *Bryonia.*

Nausea

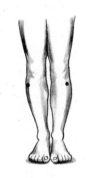

Acupressure Point: 4 fingers width (patient's fingers) below the apex of the kneecap, 1 finger width to the side edge of the tibia. Press firmly with the thumb or middle finger and rotate 2 to 4 minutes.

Herbal Teas: Drink infusions of chamomile, peppermint, or ginger.

Homeopathy: After eating, *Nux vomica;* if constant, *Ipecacuanha.*

Neck Pain and Stiffness

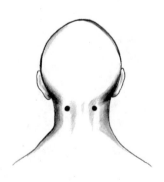

Acupressure Point I: Just below the lower edge of the skull, to the side of the depressions on both sides. Press and rotate 2 to 3 minutes, both sides.

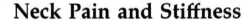

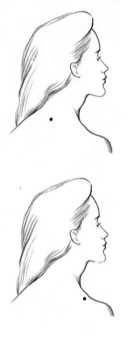

Acupressure Point II: At the space between the C-7 and T-1 dorsal spinal processes. (The C-7 vertebra is the one that protrudes when the head is bent slightly forward. T-1 is immediately below it.) Use thumb to press and rotate 2 to 3 minutes.

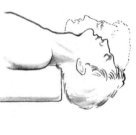

Acupressure Points III: On the hump of the shoulder, on the same vertical line as the nipple. Use thumbs or index fingers; press and rotate 2 to 3 minutes. Both shoulders.

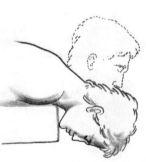

The Head Throw: Lying supine, take a few deep breaths until you are breathing rhythmically, and then allow the head to hang over the edge of the bed as illustrated. Raise the head only, using neck muscles only (do not raise chest or shoulders), then let the head fall back gently. Repeat 6 times. Turning over to a prone position, again permit the head to hang over the edge of the bed with the chin just touching the mattress. Again raise the head only (leaving the shoulders on the bed), and after raising, permit the head to fall forward to starting position. Repeat 6 times. (This exercise done regularly in the morning and at night is a useful strategy for *preventing* chronic neck stiffness. This exercise is *not* recommended for those who have had spinal surgery, radical mastectomy, or head or neck surgery.)

Yogic Neck Roll: Either sitting in a comfortable position or while standing in a shower with hot water playing on the neck and back, rotate the head toward the right shoulder as far as possible, keeping the shoulders relaxed and motionless. Then bending the neck back, rotate the head to the left shoulder as far as possible. Now turn the head forward to the center and let it drop limply. Repeat 4 or 5 times, alternately left and right direction.

Homeopathy: *Arnica montana* may relieve neck pain or soreness from overexertion.

Nosebleed

Acupressure Point: Midway between the fourth and fifth fingers, 1 finger width below the skin crease at the base of the fingers. Use fingernail to press very hard for 1 to 2 minutes. Both hands.

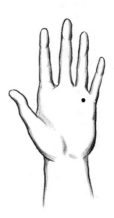

Home Remedy: Insert into the bleeding nostril a wad of cotton wool soaked in the juice of a fresh lemon.

General:
◆ Eating oranges, tomatoes, and other fruits may help to strengthen the veins so that the nose bleeds less.
◆ Almost every folk tradition includes advice to use cold objects in treating nosebleeds. For instance, in England a common prescription is to "place cold keys over the nose and

the nose at the collar level, putting the feet simultaneously in hot water." Another English idea is to "raise the arm of the side from which bleeding occurs above the head, and apply something cold to the spine." In many Latin American countries children are taught that "a cold coin on the forehead" will stop a nosebleed, while the mountain people of the southern United States have dozens of similar folk remedies, including the advice to "place a nickel under the nose between the upper lip and the gum, and press tightly." (That same prescription, but using cold bacon instead of a coin, is found in many Canadian folk traditions.)

◆ Good advice from *Where There Is No Doctor: The Village Health Care Handbook:* "In older persons especially, bleeding may come from the back part of the nose and cannot be stopped by pinching it. In this case, have the person hold a cork, corn cob, or other similar object between his teeth and, leaning forward, sit quietly and try not to swallow until the bleeding stops." (The cork keeps him from swallowing, giving the blood a chance to clot.)

Homeopathy: Phosphorus.

Poison Ivy

Home Remedies: Immediately following exposure, wash affected parts thoroughly with brown laundry soap (not detergent) and water.

Herbs and Plants: The juice from *Aloe vera* or the crushed leaves of plantain or jewelweed (which usually grows near poison ivy) are effective against the itching. Plantain is found readily in city as well as rural areas.

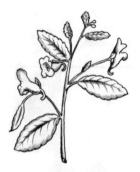

Jewelweed

Shock

Acupressure Point: Just above the middle of the depression on the surface of the upper lip, one third down from the base of the nose, two thirds up from the top edge of the upper lip. Use the thumbnail or index finger and press hard.

Homeopathy: *Arnica* every fifteen minutes; if there is agitation or restlessness, *Aconitum napellus*.

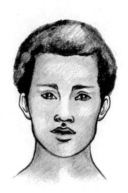

Sinusitis

Acupressure Point: Midway between the eyebrows, on the bridge of the nose. Pinch firmly and repeat for 2 to 3 minutes. (See also "Colds and Congestion.")

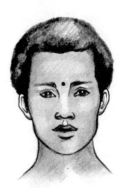

Skin Problems

Home Remedies:
♦ The juice of crushed plantain leaves may be applied locally on most skin irritations.
♦ The juice from the split leaf of the *Aloe vera* plant is helpful for a wide range of skin irritations.
♦ Alfalfa tablets are helpful in preventing eczema.
♦ For boils, apply a poultice of *chopped* garlic. Repeat until swelling has been drawn out. Do *not* lance the boil.
♦ Itching: Apply pure fresh lemon juice to the affected areas. Repeat as needed. Also

cornstarch combined with castor oil into a paste will relieve itching.

◆ For rashes, dry cornstarch makes a useful baby powder; oatmeal baths will relieve the sting of hives and itching and may help to quiet eczema pain. ("Aveeno" is a pharmaceutical oatmeal which dissolves easily in water, but generic oatmeal flakes may also be used.)

Homeopathy: For dry skin, *Belladonna* or *Pulsatilla;* for inflamed pustules, *Aconitum napellus;* for itching eruptions, *Sulphur.* (See also "Insect Bites and Stings.")

Sore Throat

Home Remedies:
◆ Gargle with 1 teaspoon of salt in a glass of warm water or alternate hourly a gargle of diluted fresh lemon juice (juice of ¼ lemon to 5 ounces warm water) and a gargle of black tea (e.g., orange pekoe). Continue as needed.
◆ Barley water mixed with fresh lemon juice is a soothing drink.

Herbal Treatment: A small amount of honey dissolved in the mouth occasionally, or slippery elm lozenges, can afford relief.

Splinters

Herbal Remedy: Make a strong infusion of agrimony (fresh or dried) and submerge affected part fully in mixture for 30 minutes. Splinter should then draw out easily.

Home Remedy: Place heated (not painfully hot) cup over affected area. Press the skin for 2 to 5 minutes, remove splinter with sterilized tweezers.

Sprains

Herbal Remedy:
◆ A fomentation of catnip reduces swelling caused by sprains.
◆ Poultices of comfrey leaves or roots moistened first with boiling water also relieve swelling and pain.
◆ Arnica lotion (made from pressings of the flower *Arnica montana)* is an inexpensive, readily available, and effective emollient.

Home Remedy: A mixture of olive oil and wintergreen makes a mild and helpful liniment.

Homeopathy: *Arnica montana,* internally and/or as a lotion but only on unbroken skin; for torn or wrenched tendons or ligaments, *Ruta graveolens.*

Sunburn

Home Remedies: Make a 1-quart brew of any black (nonherbal) tea, allow to cool, then soak clean cloths in the mixture and apply to the affected areas. (Leave cloths on skin until cold. Repeat as necessary.)
◆ The juice from the split leaf of the *Aloe vera* plant soothes and heals. Apply as often as necessary.

Toothache

Acupressure Point I: Over the back of the hand between the thumb and first finger. Massage the area with gauze-wrapped ice for seven minutes on the side corresponding to the pain site—less time if numbness sets in. Both hands.

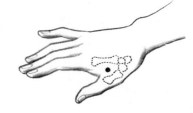

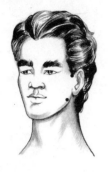

Acupressure Point II: On the jawline, about 1 finger width in front of the angle of the jawbone. Press firmly and rotate 2 to 3 minutes. Then at the depression between the upper jawbone and the edge of the ear, massage firmly with palm 2 to 3 minutes on the same side as the toothache.

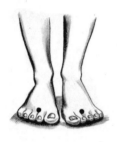

Acupressure Point III: Between the second and third toes, at the join of the metatarsals and phalanges. Press sharply with index fingernail 2 to 3 minutes.

Acupressure Point IV: At the corner of the fingernail of the index finger. Use thumbnail of other hand to press and rotate gently for 2 to 3 minutes.

Herbal Remedies:
◆ Mix 1 teaspoon of myrrh powder and 1 teaspoon boric acid in 1 pint of boiling water. Let stand for 30 minutes. Use as a gargle for inflammation of the mouth, throat, or gums.
◆ To relieve persistent bleeding after an extraction, wrap a teabag in a gauze pad, wet it, and hold against the bleeding area.

Home Remedies:
◆ A clove or oil of clove held against the tooth relieves pain. Cloves may also be mixed with water to make a tea or gargle.
◆ Half a clove of garlic, placed between the gums, will often relieve toothache.

PROMOTIVE TECHNIQUES

The following pages contain a number of exercises and techniques drawn from the other medicines that can help you develop and maintain a number of desirable conditions, ranging from improved muscle tone to deep relaxation. In addition, there are simple introductions to a number of systems that have become popular with those interested in "wellness" and "fitness," practices, such as meditation and mental imagery, that are based on the interaction of mind and body.

The Annotated Bibliography contains descriptions of a number of books that contain fuller instructions on exercises and methods that are addressed to promoting the optimal functioning of your mind and body.

Breathing Exercises

Abdominal Breathing

The "rolling breath" is effective in reducing anxiety, depression, irritability, muscular tension, and fatigue. It is also used as a part of relaxation and meditation. Read the following instructions completely before beginning to practice.

1. Lie on your back or sit in a relaxed position (as illustrated). Place one hand on your abdomen and one hand on your upper chest, below the throat. Inhale and exhale slowly, noting that the breathing normally takes place in your chest, and that the hand on your abdomen is not moved by either the inhalation or the exhalation.

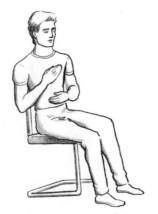

2. Now breathe in slowly *through the nose,* filling your abdomen and lowering your diaphragm. After your abdomen is filled and expanded, complete the breath by continuing to

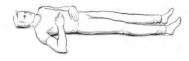

inhale, filling your chest with air and raising it. (It may be helpful to imagine that you are inflating a balloon in your abdomen.)

3.   Exhale slowly and completely from your upper chest, then from your abdomen. Repeat several times.

4. With practice and concentration, the breathing will become rhythmical and rolling. It will feel like a wave, beginning in the abdomen, moving upward to your chest, relaxing in the chest, and then returning to the abdomen. You may mentally count as follows:

—inhale into the abdomen   1-2-3-4
—inhale into the chest   5-6-7-8
—hold   1-2-3
—exhale from the chest   1-2-3-4
—exhale from the abdomen   5-6-7-8
—hold   1-2-3
—repeat

With practice, the periods of inhalation, exhalation, and holds will lengthen. Always exhale very completely.

After the breathing has been learned, it may no longer be necessary to put your hands on your abdomen and chest. The breathing, once learned, can also be done standing up—in the supermarket line, for example, or anytime nervousness or tension begins, reversing the usual pattern in which tension results in even more shallow breathing.

The Complete Breath

Complete Yogic breathing is beneficial for many of the same conditions as the abdominal breathing described above, but it is slightly more complex and difficult to learn. It consists of three parts: the low, abdominal breath; a middle breath; and the upper chest breath. Again, before beginning, read the instructions through completely and then follow each step as it is described.

1.   Lie on your back with legs bent and the soles of your feet flat on the floor.

2.   Slowly inhale through your nose, inflating your abdomen, being conscious of the abdominal muscles. Repeat several times.

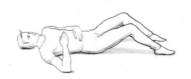

3.   Still lying on your back, inhale slowly through your nose, concentrating on your ribs and expanding them sideways. To demonstrate this, place your hands on your sides over the ribs. Neither your abdomen nor your chest should move during the middle breath. Repeat several times. (This is often the most difficult part to learn.)

4.   Now practice the upper chest breath, slowly lifting your collarbone and shoulders. Repeat several times.

5.   When the separate parts are learned, combine them into a rolling, wavelike breath as in the abdominal breathing. Repeat several times.

The Energizing Breath

This exercise is sometimes called "skull shining," since it energizes and brings a sense of radiant brightness to your head. It is accomplished in merely three steps:

1.   While standing or sitting, inhale deeply through your nose and press your lips close to your teeth, leaving only a narrow slit between them.

2.   Exhale forcefully through the slit in a series of short, distinct bursts of air.

3.   After exhaling all the air, take several relaxed deep breaths, and repeat once or twice more.

The Warming (or Cooling) Breath

1.   Sit or stand quietly and get into the rhythm of the rolling breath.

2.   Continue the breathing. Visualize, in your

mind's eye, a perforated tube running through the center of your body from head to pelvis. This "tube" permits air to be channeled into all parts of your body—out through your shoulders, along your arms, and into your hands, through your hips, down your legs, and into your feet. Visualize, with each deep exhalation, the part of the breath that is moving through the openings to the outer extremities. Feel it as gentle air, sending warmth to the ends of your fingers and toes.

3. Continue breathing in deeply, sending warm exhaled breath to all the parts of you that are chilled. Continue this regular in-out breathing, increasing the warmth with each breath. (Obviously, the same exercise can be used for cooling simply by visualizing cold, instead of hot, air.)

Total Body Relaxation

1. Clench one fist as hard as possible and then let go. Do this several times to make sure that the difference between *tension* and *relaxation* is clear. Notice also the difference in feeling between the clenched-fist arm and the other one.

2. Lying (or seated) comfortably, with your eyes closed, do abdominal or complete breathing. (See pp. 181–183.)

3. You will tense, then let go, each part of your body, starting at the feet and working up to the face and scalp. As you do this, tell yourself, "I am relaxing my feet . . . my calves," and so on. Let all other thoughts drift by.

4. Breathe in and out through your nose. Take deep, regular breaths, emptying your lungs each time you exhale. Your breathing will become slow and rhythmical.

5. Now begin with your feet. Tense . . . tense . . . tense . . . let go!

6. Next do your calves, your lower legs. Tense . . . tense . . . tense . . . let go!

7. Now the knees and thighs. Tense . . .

tense . . . tense . . . let go!

8. Now the buttocks and genitals. Tense . . . tense . . . tense . . . let go!

9. Now the lower abdomen. Tense . . . tense . . . tense . . . let go!

10. Now the chest. Tense . . . tense . . . tense . . . let go!

11. Now the back. Tense . . . tense . . . tense . . . let go!

12. Now the hands and wrist. Tense . . . tense . . . tense . . . let go!

13. Now the upper arms and shoulders. Tense . . . tense . . . tense . . . let go!

14. Now the neck. Tense . . . tense . . . tense . . . let go!

15. Now relax your jaw, let it drop. Now "scrunch up" your whole face, your mouth, cheeks, eyes, forehead and scalp. Tense . . . tense . . . tense . . . let go!

16. With practice, you will achieve deep relaxation easily. Once this skill is acquired, you can do it while sitting in a chair or during a short break in your work.

Meditation

Hundreds of books have been written on the technique of meditation, covering not only the spiritual implications of the practice, but some of the ways the technique can be useful for maintaining or improving one's health. Some of these books are described in the Annotated Bibliography. But for those who have never attempted to use meditative practice, the following simple introductory exercise will give you a flavor of the experience.

1. Choose as quiet a place as possible.

2. Choose a comfortable position, one that you can hold for about twenty minutes, either sitting in a chair or tailor-fashion on the floor.

3. Choose something to dwell on—a word or sound. (Herbert Benson and Miriam Klipper, in their book *The Relaxation Response,* recommend repetition of the word "one".)

4.   Adopt a passive attitude, letting thoughts which come to mind simply slide by without the customary "latching on" to them.

5.   After settling into the chosen position, scan your body for tension, or do the relaxation exercise, tensing and relaxing the body parts from feet to the head. (See instructions on p. 184.)

6.   Breathing through the nose slowly and rhythmically, become aware of your breath. Repeat the chosen word or sound each time you exhale. Let thoughts simply slide by.

7.   Continue for fifteen minutes. Do not use an alarm clock, but you may keep a clock or watch handy to check with. In meditation one loses track of the time, but usually people automatically return to the regular conscious state in about fifteen minutes.

8.   Practice this technique at least five times a week for a month before deciding to continue or discontinue.

"Palming"

This is a simple exercise to help rest and refresh your eyes and mind, especially during extended periods of reading.

1.   Briskly rub your hands together to warm them.

2.   Close your eyes and place your cupped hands over them gently. The heels of your hand should be flat on your cheekbones, while the center of your palms should be over your eyes, arched over your eyelids.

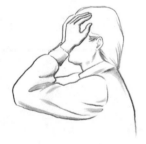

3.   Try to keep your back straight while "palming," perhaps by resting your elbows on the back of a chair during the exercise.

4.   Do this for five minutes, repeat as often as needed.

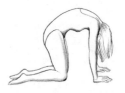

"The Cat"

This is a simple exercise based on Yogic principles. It helps to exercise the spine and abdomen, and is particularly helpful for women after childbirth.

1. Get on to your hands and knees, imagining that you are a beautiful cat with a very long, furry tail. Now, with your head down, round your back and droop your tail down. (Really feel that tail!)

2. Then raise your head up, arch your back, and raise your tail as you exhale.

3. Inhale, moving the tail down; exhale, moving the tail up. (Remember: Don't move your head, just your tail.)

4. Now make a few circles with your cat's tail.

5. Repeat the sequence five or six times.

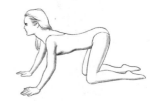

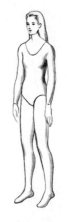

"Picking Grapes"

This simple stretching exercise will help you achieve increased flexibility, and it is especially helpful for older people because it emphasizes no special straining.

1. Stand with your feet separated about the width of your shoulders, and stay for a few moments with your knees unlocked and your body in as relaxed a state as possible.

2. When you feel that you are totally relaxed, let your body fall forward from your waist, making no attempt to touch the ground but with your fingers outstretched toward the ground, still in as relaxed a manner as possible.

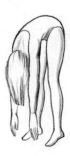

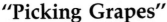

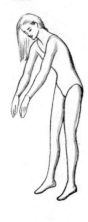

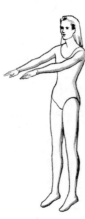

3. Then slowly and rhythmically rise from the bent position, allowing your upper torso to follow the lead of your arms as they ascend and eventually reach toward the sky.

4. At the point when your arms are extended as far as possible, stand up on your tiptoes, begin to wiggle all your fingers, and reach toward an imaginary grape arbor as if you were picking the fruit off the vine. Move around if it will make you feel more comfortable and balanced. Feel your spine and back being gently arched and stretched, and that your hips are rolled back, with your face looking upward as the fingers "pluck the grapes."

5. After several moments in this outstretched position, slowly permit your upper torso once again to fall forward, with the hands, head, and shoulders descending to the floor.

6. After a few moments in the bent position, raise up your torso and arms, and allow your body to stretch up fully, rise up on your toes, and repeat the "picking of the grapes."

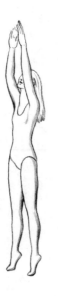

"The Turtle"

This simple exercise is an adaptation of an ancient Chinese Yogic practice. It is designed to help you relax your neck and shoulder muscles and to release the tension and tiredness that so often occur in the neck and back.

1.   Sitting or standing in a relaxed position, slowly let your chin fall onto your chest. You will feel the back of your neck and top of your head stretching upward and your shoulders relaxing downward as you do this.

2.   Now move your head back, bringing the back of your skull down as if you were trying to touch the back of your neck with your head.

3.   With your head pulled back in this way, pull your shoulders up on both sides, as though you were trying to touch your ears with them.

4.   Do all these movements slowly, inhaling as you stretch your head back, exhaling as you let it fall to your chest.

5.   Do this several times each morning and before going to bed, or anytime you feel tension in your neck or shoulders.

"Bozo the Clown"

You may remember that Bozo is the weighted toy that children hit, which returns to an upright position because it is filled with sand on the bottom. The exercise based on this toy is intended to encourage stability and balance when you are walking by reinforcing your consciousness of your pelvis and its connection as the major link between your legs and your upper torso.

1. Sit on the floor comfortably, as cross-legged as possible.

2. Close your eyes and breathe deeply, imagining the breath coming from the base of the spine.

3. Then, exhaling, imagine the breath to be moving down the back of the spine. Feel a floating sensation with each exhalation.

4. Move the head several times nodding "yes" (forward and back), "no" (turning the head from side to side), and "maybe" (tilting the head from one shoulder to the other).

5. Try to feel as centered and bottom-heavy as possible. Feel that a large weight, just below the navel, is weighing you down. Now lean forward slowly, continuing to feel that centered weight. Rock slowly back to center.

6. Now lean to the right, feeling the weight just below the navel. Return to center.

7. Now lean to the left, feeling the weight in the pelvic area. Return to center.

8. Gently move around in a circle. Always return to the center, upright position, feeling that a special weight is keeping you balanced.

9. Now stand, close your eyes, and imagine once again the feeling you experienced while leaning and rocking on the floor. This exercise attempts to encourage the subjective feeling that the center of gravity is actually low in the body, just above the genitals, and not mentally held in your head, chest, or throat.

10. After a few moments of deep breathing and recollection of the weighted feeling in the pelvis, walk very slowly back and forth and around the room.

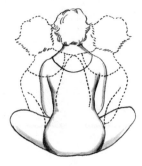

Self-massage

Throughout this massage, close your eyes and concentrate on the feeling in your fingers, skin, and body. Breathe deeply and slowly.

1. Begin by tapping the top of your head gently with your fingertips. Let your fingers dance around all over your skull.

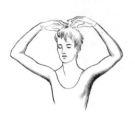

2. With the tips of your fingers, begin to massage your ears, starting with the top rim and circling your entire ear.

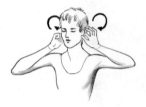

3. When your fingers approach your earlobes, massage gently in a circular way. Let your fingers move to the indentations right behind your ear. Do a slow circular massage on these indentations.

4. Gently rub your neck muscles from the base of your skull downward.

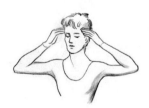

5. Move your hands around to your face. Pull your forehead horizontally from the midline to the side, running your hands along your forehead in a gentle movement from side to side.

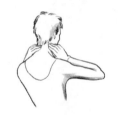

6. Massage around the sinuses and the bony orbit of your eyes (be sure not to massage your eyeballs).

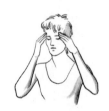

7. Use your fingertips to massage the sides of the tip of your nose.

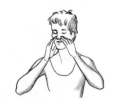

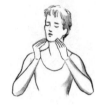

8. Move your fingers in a circular motion on your jawbones, coming forward slowly from your ears down to your chin.

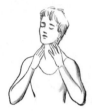

9. When you come to the tip of your chin, use your hands to pull downwards gently on the front of your neck.

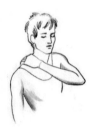

10. Crossing your left hand over your body, massage your right shoulder muscles vigorously, keeping the other arm and hand tucked behind you to support your back. Do the same for your left shoulder with your right hand. Knead your shoulders, particularly in back and toward the neck.

Foot Massage

Foot massage can help stimulate every organ in the body and can help to relieve tension and regulate digestion. It is particularly useful for the relief of headache.

Though there is some controversy as to whether the "reflex areas" defined in "Foot Reflexology" are as specific as shown on the charts on the next page, a soothing foot massage is beneficial to give or to receive.

Use a few drops of vegetable oil, an aloe gel, or other light lotion. Massage both feet firmly, top and bottom, and gently twist and stretch each toe. Continue for up to, but not longer than, fifteen minutes.

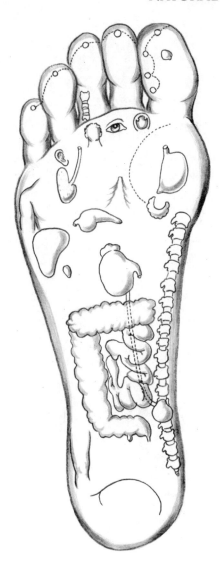
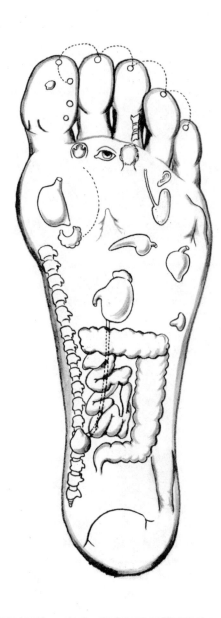

ANNOTATED
BIBLIOGRAPHY

Acupuncture Anesthesia. Bethesda, Md.: National Institute of Health, 1975. The translation of a Chinese publication of the same title. This is a technical manual for physicians, but has been one of the influential publications in the legitimization of acupuncture in the West.

Albright, Peter, and Albright, Bets Parker, eds. *Body, Mind, and Spirit.* Brattleboro, Vt.: Stephen Greene Press, 1980. A somewhat ecstatic collection of essays that argues for a unity of the "triune" aspects of human nature. Heavy emphasis on a "natural" approach to birth, yoga, meditation, self-healing, herbs, biofeedback, kinesiology, Oriental medicine, and reflexology. Insistent in tone, but useful as a survey of parts of the holistic movement in medicine and health.

Alexander, Franz. *Psychosomatic Medicine: Its Principles and Applications.* New York: W. W. Norton & Co., 1950. Alexander was one of the Freudian-trained pioneers who elaborated on the connection between mind and body, especially in diagnosing illness. His work is the most influential of the early works that legitimizes psychosomatic principle, though the reverse of the principle—that mind could work to cure body illness—was not addressed until much later, when it was seen to be a revival of ancient principles.

Arano, Luisa Cogliati. *The Medieval Health Handbook: Tacuinum Sanitatis.* New York: George Braziller, 1976. Published as an artistic artifact, but instructive on the history of the use of herbs and dietary advice for better health. Beautifully printed and rewarding to read as a piece of historical continuity.

Baïracli-Levy, Juliette de. *Common Herbs for Natural Health.* New York: Schocken Books, 1973. A small but useful herbal, with particularly clear illustrations and a good assortment of specific remedies.

Barlow, Wilfred. *The Alexander Technique.* New York: Alfred A. Knopf, 1979. The best general introduction to the system of "reorganizing the economy of the body" developed by F. Matthias Alexander. This method has survived and flourished for almost a hundred years, and a reading of its principles will explain this success, though reading alone cannot replace at least some workshop experience.

Bennett, Hal Zina. *Cold Comfort.* New York: Clarkson Potter, 1979. A whole book about one of the most common afflictions besetting the human race, this slim and readable volume is especially noteworthy because it gives as much attention to nontraditional cures as to the established therapies. Handy.

Benson, Herbert. *The Relaxation Response.* New York: Avon Books, 1976. Now a near classic, this book summarizes Benson's early work in converting some of the principles of Transcendental Meditation (TM) to a simpler technique for relaxation that is particularly suitable for the stressed Westerner. A remarkably helpful book, introducing the reader to relaxation exercises that are now generally credited with helping patients with hypertension, chronic headache, gastrointestinal disorders, back pain, and other stress-related conditions.

Bergson, Anika, and Tuchak, Vladimir. *Shiatzu.* New York: Pinnacle Books, 1976. Much shorter and less comprehensive than the Ohashi book. This is a straightforward first aid manual based on Shiatsu principles. Handy, but not illuminating.

Blake, Michael. *The Natural Healer's Acupressure Book.* New York: Holt, Rinehart & Winston, 1977. Of the many manuals teaching variations and adaptations of classical Chinese acupressure techniques, this is one of the best. Clearly written and illustrated, its description of GJo techniques is helpful to practitioners and laymen alike.

Bleything, Dennis, and Dawson, Ron. *Primitive Medical Aid in the Wilderness.* Beaverton, Ore.: Wilderness Is . . . , 1971. A compact pocket guide intended originally for serious hikers and backpackers, but useful for city or suburban situations requiring quick, improvisational aid using common plants and ordinary household materials.

Bloomfield, H. H. and Kory, R. B. *The Holistic Way to Health and Happiness.* New York: Simon & Schuster, 1978. Billed as a general survey of the application of holistic principles in general medical practice, the main emphasis throughout is on the virtue of Transcendental Meditation as a help in dealing with stress reactions.

Bricklin, Mark. *The Practical Encyclopedia of Natural Healing.* Emmaus, Pa.: Rodale Press, 1976. Fulfills its title in comprehensiveness and, as with most books from Rodale, can be trusted as having useful and effective information, albeit from the strong bias of the "organic" and "natural" food and vitamin movement.

Brody, Howard. *Ethical Decision in Medicine.* Boston: Little, Brown & Co., 1976. A wide-ranging book on many aspects of medicine and the doctor-patient relationship. Particularly noteworthy for Brody's original definition of human health as the systems-rooted impact of man on environment and environment's influence on man.

Brown, Barbara. *New Mind, New Body.* New York: Bantam Books, 1975. One of the classics in the field, this book is a clear and convincing presentation not only of biofeedback but also of the principle of self-regulation that characterizes other systems. Best read along with the Greens' *Beyond Biofeedback.*

————. *Stress and the Art of Biofeedback.* New York: Harper & Row Publishers, 1977. An extension of her earlier work, this book concentrates on the application of clinical biofeedback training to stress-related conditions such as hypertension, asthma, and cardiovascular conditions. Authoritative and impressive.

Burang, Theodore. *The Tibetan Art of Healing.* London: Watkins & Co., 1973. One of the few books available in English that summarizes the general principles of Tibetan medicine, including herbs, nutrition, and the unique Tibetan version of the humoral theory of disease. Brief, but useful.

Cannon, W. B. *The Wisdom of the Body.* New York: W. W. Norton & Co., 1939. A pioneer work, now endlessly cited, emphasizing the inextricable relationship between mind and body and the equally circular relationship between physical and emotional health. Almost a "holy" book to holistic practitioners, but useful now mainly for its historical interest.

Capra, Fritjof. *The Tao of Physics.* Boulder, Colo.: Shambhala Publications, 1975. Addresses many issues of this book—parallels in Eastern and Western thought, the uses of paradox, and the need for universalizing human knowledge—by relating various forms of Eastern mysticism to the findings and speculations of modern physics.

Carlson, Rick J. *The End of Medicine.* New York: John Wiley & Sons, 1975. A general critique of the whole health care system and the practice of medicine, much more balanced in tone and context than Illich. One of the first clear statements of the need for a system oriented toward prevention and promotive medicine rather than merely curative technology.

Chan, Pedro. *Finger Acupressure.* New York: Ballantine Books, 1976. A brief, clearly photographed guide to some basic acupressure points for first aid relief.

Chang, Stephen Thomas. *The Book of Internal Exercises.* San Francisco: Strawberry Hill Press, 1978. An impressive manual of instruction for exercises drawn from the Taoist Yogic teachings of ancient China. These noncalisthenic techniques combine mind and body disciplines in a way that can be unusually helpful in the relief of symptomatic complaints ranging from headaches to arthritis, but their main value is in enhancing health.

————. *The Complete Book of Acupuncture.* Millbrae, Calif.: Celestial Arts, 1976. Particularly recommended for laymen and physicians, because it goes far beyond its title to present one of the most accessible summaries of the philosophical and psychological background of all of Chinese medicine. Includes detailed instructions for treating forty-eight specific ailments. Clearly written and well illustrated.

Coon, Nelson. *Using Plants for Healing.* Emmaus, Pa.: Rodale Press, 1979. An "underground" classic, first published in 1963, covering almost every aspect of the healing properties of plants: history, preparation of medicinal plants, and a comprehensive descriptive guide of hundreds of plants for everyday use. Straightforward, authoritative, and useful.

Coulter, Harris L. *Homeopathic Medicine.* St. Louis, Mo.: Formur International, 1972. The best brief introduction to homeopathy.

————. *Divided Legacy.* Washington, D.C.: Wehawken Book Co., 1973. A dense, three-volume history of medicine, with a scholarly emphasis on the schism that has divided the field since ancient times. Extremely worthwhile for any serious student, physician, or researcher in holistic health.

————. *Homeopathic Science and Modern Medicine.* Richmond, Calif.: North Atlantic Books, 1981. This general introduction to the history and theoretical basis of homeopathy is totally accessible to patients as well as physicians. Valuable.

Cousins, Norman. *Anatomy of an Illness.* New York: W. W. Norton & Co., 1979. Not just a bestselling profile of one man's "miracle cure," but also a serious examination of continuing issues in medical treatment: vitamin C, patient self-management, the holistic health movement, etc. Cousins is an inordinately literate, clear, and felicitous writer.

Cummings, Stephen, and Ullman, Dana. *Everybody's Guide to Homeopathic Medicines.* Los Angeles: Jeremy P. Tarcher, Inc., 1984. Easy to read for its clear presentation of the history and theory of homeopathy, this book is equally easy to use for its accessible guide to remedies. A real contribution.

Davis, Martha, and McKay, Matthew. *The Relaxation and Stress Reduction Workbook.* San Francisco: New Harbinger Publications, 1980. A current manual of instructions and exercises—well-illustrated—in progressive relaxation (the system first developed by Edmund Jacobson), with special emphasis on the application of muscle relaxation for stress-related illnesses. Extremely useful for laymen as well as for the health care professionals for whom it was written.

Dawson, Adele. *Health, Happiness, and the Pursuit of Herbs.* Brattleboro, Vt.: Stephen Greene Press, 1980. Despite the coy title, this is one of the most valuable books in the field. Covers growing and drying of herbs as well as an interesting history of medicinal and culinary uses of herbs through the ages. Arranged by seasons for practical guidance. A valuable delight.

De Langre, Jacques. *Do-in Two.* 2nd. ed. Magalia, Calif.: Happiness Press, 1978. An almost manic potpourri about the occult or esoteric roots of the theory of the life-force. Imbedded in this free-form mosaic are some truly interesting and valuable procedures that combine self-massage with acupressure.

Densmore, Frances. *How Indians Use Wild Plants for Food, Medicine, and Crafts.* New York: Dover Publications, 1974. A facsimile of a portion of the Forty-fourth Annual Report of the Bureau of American Ethnology 1926–1971, this work covers more than the medicinal use of herbs, and the text devoted to healing plants demonstrates the remarkably wide-ranging pharmacopeia developed by Native Americans.

Dintenfass, Julius. *Chiropractic: A Modern Way to Health.* New York: Harcourt Brace Jovanovich, 1971. A good introduction to the principles of the chiropractic approach to preventive and curative manipulation of the spine as it is generally practiced in the United States.

Dossey, Larry. *Space, Time, and Medicine.* Boulder, Colo.: Shambhala Publications, 1982. An imaginative and speculative book that brings the current critique of medicine to the area of "new physics." This book does not follow the holistic "party line," but rather suggests that new ways of looking at the brain, at the concept of time, and at consciousness itself can bring on the next and needed stage of medical theory and practice. Original and important.

Downing, George. *The Massage Book.* New York: Random House, 1978. One of the books that helped launch the era of the "sensual massage," this book is a delightful introduction to the useful techniques of "amateur" massages for health.

Dubos, René. *Man Adapting.* New Haven: Yale University Press, 1965. One of several comprehensive views of human nature and environment by the late, distinguished philosopher and scientist. Though the factual content relates to the mechanism of "adaptation," this book also contains the seeds of Dubos's positive interest in the possibility of increased self-regulation of body, mind, and spirit. A superb book.

————. *Man, Medicine, and Environment.* New York: New American Library, 1968. One of the keystone works in the development of the new field of "human ecology," a perspective that defines human health as the response of mankind to the worlds of nature, thought, feeling, and technology. Medicine, in this view, becomes potentially the great catalytic force in advancing not only the health of human beings, but also the understanding of the action of those beings.

————. *The Mirage of Health.* Garden City, N.Y.: Doubleday & Co., 1959. One of the books that established the author as one of the most influential thinkers on the subjects of health, illness, medicine, and the environment. Written almost thirty years ago, the ideas are still astonishingly fresh and, regrettably, still not heeded as seriously as they deserve to be.

Durckheim, Karlfried. *Hara: The Vital Centre of Man.* London: George Allen & Unwin, 1971. A thoughtful and gracefully written explication of the principle of "centering," especially as found in Japanese religion and philosophy. Includes descriptions of exercises in breathing, sitting, walking, and habits of posture.

Eliade, Mircea. *Patanjali and Yoga.* New York: Schocken Books, 1975. A clear and fascinating look at the history, development, and meaning of the Yogic tradition. Focuses on the *Yoga Sutras* of Patanjali, the first codification of the principles of "classic Yoga." Important.

Erickson, Milton H., and Rossi, Ernest L. *Experiencing Hypnosis.* New York: Irvington House, 1976. One of the best books depicting the theory and practice of the innovative Milton H. Erickson, who launched a new era in hypnotherapy.

Feldenkrais, Moshe. *Awareness Through Movement.* New York: Harper & Row Publishers, 1972. Not a substitute for the actual experiences of Feldenkrais's exercises, which are remarkably effective, but a comfortable introduction to his theories regarding posture, breathing, coordination of movements, self-image, and—most important—the connection between thinking and moving. Twelve exercises are described in detail, in addition to basic theories. Important, because Feldenkrais is so important.

Forgey, William W. *Wilderness Medicine.* Pittsboro, Ind.: Indiana Camp Supply Books, 1979. Medicine and the ways of the wilderness are combined here by a physician devoted to both. Some medical advice and instructions are mixed with helpful improvisational procedures for emergencies and good counsel for people going on an overnight hike or a serious expedition.

Foster, Gertrude B. *Herbs for Every Garden.* New York: E. P. Dutton, 1963. Though only modestly devoted to the curative power of plants, this book is one of the most straightforward and unintimidating guides to growing herbs of all kinds. Indispensable if you want to grow your own—indoors, in the city, or in a spacious garden.

Frank, Jerome D. *Persuasion and Healing.* 2nd ed. Baltimore: Johns Hopkins University Press, 1973. A book that has inspired a whole generation of others who deal with the power of the mind to aid in killing or curing human beings. Especially important for its emphasis on the importance of the belief systems of both patient and healer in the therapeutic encounter. Immensely readable, and basic to any serious study of the mind-body relationship.

Friedman, Meyer, and Rosenman, Ray H. *Type A Behavior and Your Heart.* New York: Alfred A. Knopf, 1979. The book that established a personality profile that was as predictive of coronary trouble as the other big three indicators—smoking, serum cholesterol, and hypertension. Particularly influential in legitimizing the new field of "behavioral medicine," a Western approach to respecting the effect of internal states and attitudes on biochemical processes.

Gibson, D. M. *First Aid Homeopathy in Accidents and Ailments.* 4th ed. London: British Homeopathic Association, 1975. The closest thing to an official homeopathic first aid manual, this guide covers recommended prescriptions for afflictions ranging from abscesses to wounds, and includes treatment for many internal ailments as well. Authoritative, direct, and useful.

Goldstein, Kurt. *Human Nature in the Light of Psychopathology.* New York: Schocken Books, 1966. The book that revived Smuts's idea of holism, and applied it to the concept of self-actualization. Goldstein's work inspired Abraham Maslow, one of the fathers of humanistic psychology, which in turn spawned the holistic health movement. An important book.

Gordon, James, and Rosenthal, Raymond. *The Healing Partnership.* Washington: Aurora Associates, 1984. A group of four impressive essays on the need for an approach to both medical training and medical care that gives equal importance to health education, complementary medical practices, and patient self-management.

Gordon, Richard. *Your Healing Hands.* Santa Cruz, Calif.: Unity Press, 1978. A modest introduction to "polarity energy balancing," an extension of the polarity therapy system developed by Dr. Randolph Stone. Sometimes the lyricism of "healing" obscures the content of the quite beneficial techniques.

Graedon, Joe. *The People's Pharmacy.* New York: Avon Books, 1979. One of the dozens of books rolling off the presses that debunk or attack synthetic drugs. I have found this the most useful, because it is not hysterical or excessive. A good guide to what really happens when you ingest those "miracles."

Green, Elmer, and Green, Alyce. *Beyond Biofeedback.* New York: Dell Publishing Co., 1977. Two distinguished researchers demonstrate here not only the principles of gaining voluntary control of internal states, but relate the development of Western technological approaches to the traditional disciplines of Hindu medicine that can also bear on modern health and self-care.

Griggs, Barbara. *Green Pharmacy.* New York: Viking Press, 1982. A delightfully written history of herbs that surrounds a well-stated and persuasive case for a return to plant-based medicine. Most impressive.

Grossinger, Richard. *Planet Medicine: From Stone Age Shamanism to Post-Industrial Healing.* Garden City, N.Y.: Anchor Press/Doubleday, 1980. A remarkable book that looks at not only the history of medicine but at the deeper anthropological and psychocultural roots of the ideas of healing that have appeared all across human history. In both its factual and speculative content it is brilliant and original, and should be read by anyone with a genuine interest in the evolution of medicine and its connection with the language, the arts, and the behavior of all recorded cultures.

Gunther, Bernard. *Sense Relaxation.* New York: Macmillan Publishing Co., 1974. One of the earliest and most successful books addressed to sensory awareness, the wedding of consciousness to body states so as to enhance control of both. Beautifully, if not downright romantically, photographed, the book is a gentle primer on gentle self-control.

Haich, Elisabeth, and Yesudian, Selva Raja. *Yoga and Health.* New York: Harper & Row Publishers, 1972. A brief but extremely useful manual of breathing and movement exercises.

Hand, Wayland D., ed. *American Folk Medicine.* Berkeley and Los Angeles: University of California Press, 1976. A valuable collection of papers arising from an important 1973 conference. Presentations include ancient and modern folk medicine and medical beliefs, and the cultural mix includes Amish, Cajun, Jamaican, Mexican-American and American Indian practices. Fascinating.

Hanna, Thomas. *The Body of Life.* New York: Alfred A. Knopf, 1980. An exceptionally literate and sensitive examination of the functional integration system of Moshe Feldenkrais, with relevant excursions into the work of other great teachers of somatic awareness such as F. Matthias Alexander and Charlotte Selver. Particularly useful in understanding the theory and mechanics of reeducating the body to move efficiently and freely.

Hastings, Arthur; Fadiman, James; and Gordon, James, eds. *Health for the Whole Person,* Boulder, Colo.: Westview Press, 1980. Subtitled *The Complete Guide to Holistic Medicine,* the book is a collection of essays and annotated bibliographies on subjects ranging from medical self-care to oral health and dentistry, from hypnosis to homeopathy. Useful survey by distinguished contributors, including Herbert Benson, Joe Kamiya, David Cheek, Harris Coulter, and others.

Hewitt, James. *The Complete Yoga Book.* New York: Schocken Books, 1978. A 550-page encyclopedia, consolidating three books on the Yoga of posture, the Yoga of breathing, and the Yoga of meditation by an English author of more than twenty books on Yoga and associated subjects. Comprehensive and contemporary.

Hill, Ann, ed. *A Visual Encyclopedia of Unconventional Medicine.* New York: Crown Publishers, 1978. Originally published in Great Britain (and therefore including information about systems more popular there such as color therapy, radionics, etc.) This is an interesting symposium of articles on dozens of unorthodox systems, from acupuncture to radiesthesia. Well illustrated, but the directory of referrals for further information will benefit only residents of the United Kingdom.

Hippocrates. *Hippocrates.* Translated by W. H. S. Jones. Cambridge: Harvard University Press, 1923. The standard English translation of the works of the "father of medicine." Interesting not only for the aphoristic wisdom that seems so timeless, but also as an introduction to principles that have governed the practice of medicine for centuries.

Huang, Al Chung-liang. *Embrace Tiger, Return to Mountain.* New York: Bantam Books, 1978. Not intended as a manual of instruction in T'ai Chi, this is nevertheless the best introduction to the spirit of the Chinese meditation-in-motion system, and provides an easy access to the Taoist attitudes that also govern much of Chinese medicine.

Hyatt, Richard. *Chinese Herbal Medicine.* New York: Schocken Books, 1978. A literate and fascinating small volume that covers history and theory as well as practical prescriptions for Chinese herbal remedies. Though fastidious in not claiming to be a first aid manual, this book, in informed hands, could be most useful. In any case, it makes good and provocative reading, and it includes a brief but useful directory of sources for Chinese herbs in major U.S. cities.

Illich, Ivan. *Medical Nemesis.* New York: Bantam Books, 1977. A strident and polemical critique of modern Western medicine, and particularly the overtechnologized, hospital-based health care system. Despite the tone, the arguments are persuasive and thoughtful.

Ingham, Eunice D. *Stories the Feet Can Tell Through Reflexology.* St. Petersburg, Fla.: Ingham Publishing, 1966. Originally written in 1938, this book is a sincere, homely collection of anecdotes about the success of foot reflexology (or zone therapy) in treating conditions from asthma to kidney failure. Primitive and evangelical as it is, the book is a clear introduction to this controversial therapy.

Iyengar, B. K. S. *Light on Yoga.* New York: Schocken Books, 1979. An authoritative book by a renowned teacher of Yoga (Yehudi Menuhin was one of his famous students), this book contains over six hundred photographs of Hatha Yoga postures and a clear text on the Yogic approach to health and fitness.

Jackson, Mildred, and Teague, Terri. *The Handbook to Alternatives to Clinical Medicine.* Oakland: Privately printed, 1975. A potpourri of herbal prescriptions and recipes that ranges in its specific remedies from simple sunburn to heart attacks. Grandiose in some of its claims, but useful and reasonable advice is sandwiched between the excesses.

Jacobson, Edmund. *Progressive Relaxation.* 2nd ed. Chicago: University of Chicago Press, 1938. The pioneer volume, based in part on the author's discovery that he could alleviate his own insomnia with muscle relaxation. Introduces the basic techniques of systematically tensing and relaxing whole muscle groups, a technique that has become an integral part of many newer systems including guided imagery and biofeedback training.

————. *You Must Relax.* New York: McGraw-Hill, 1978. Despite its unrelaxed title, this book, originally published in 1939, summarizes the author's important discovery of the connection between residual muscle tension and mental activities. As such, it is the keystone book in the attempt to create a Western system of self-regulation that begins to approach the ancient Yogic tradition.

Jaffe, Dennis. *Healing from Within.* New York: Alfred A. Knopf, 1980. An often moving book that demonstrates through both narrative and exercises some of the ways that patients, both individually and in groups, can engage more actively not just in the maintenance of health but in the self-treatment of illness and disability.

Jones, Frank Pierce. *Body Awareness in Action.* New York: Schocken Books, 1976. A wonderfully readable book about the Alexander technique by an important American teacher of the system who studied with F. M. and A. R. Alexander. Jones not only taught the system, he developed equipment and experiments at Tufts University that demonstrate why the relearning of posture and movement could relieve some diseases as well as provide greater stamina and a sense of well-being. Important.

Kadar, Sudir. *Shamans, Mystics, and Doctors.* New York: Alfred A. Knopf, 1982. Though primarily addressed to "mental health" as defined in both East and West, this exceptionally literate and sensitive book sheds a great deal of light on Hindu tradition and Ayurvedic medicine.

Kao, Frederick F., and Kao, John J., eds. *Chinese Medicine—New Medicine.* New York: Neale Watson Academic Publications, 1977. Published for the Institute for Advanced Research in Asian Science and Medicine, this collection of scholarly monographs ranges from general essays on history and philosophy to technical papers on jaundice. Worth reading for the brief biography of the great naturalist Li Shih-chen.

Kaptchuk, Ted W. *The Web That Has No Weaver: Understanding Chinese Medicine.* New York: Congdon & Weed, 1984. The best and most comprehensive book on the subject yet written in English, useful to the merely curious reader, but essential to the serious student. Particularly valuable for seeing the comparative ways that Western and Chinese medical theories approach disease and treatment. A remarkable achievement.

Kaslof, Leslie, ed. *Wholistic Dimensions in Healing.* Garden City, N.Y.: Doubleday & Co., 1978. A resource guide and catalogue made up of short essays on a vast range of therapeutics, including faith healing. The contributors are by and large respected authorities in their fields, and for quick information the book is immensely useful, as is the directory of resources in each subject area.

Kiev, Ari. *Magic, Faith, and Healing.* New York: Macmillan Publishing Co., 1964. One of the best explorations of the range of nonmedical healing practices throughout the world.

Kloss, Jethro. *Back to Eden.* New York: Bantam Books, 1976. Originally published in 1939, the revived paperback edition has become one of the most popular books on the healing power of herbs. The book is a compendium of natural-healing techniques of all kinds as well as a down-home health guide to exercise, fasting, and diet. Fervent and too general in many respects, it is still interesting and worthwhile.

Knowles, John, ed. *Doing Better and Feeling Worse.* New York: W. W. Norton & Co., 1977. One of the most quoted book titles in the health care field, this is a collection of critical essays by establishment figures in health and medicine, all adding up to a powerful critique of the disease orientation in modern medicine, and advocating—sometimes too shrilly—that the "right" to health care should be replaced by a "moral obligation to preserve one's own health." Of particular interest to those interested in public health policy.

Krieger, Dolores. *The Therapeutic Touch.* Englewood Cliffs, N.J.: Prentice-Hall, 1979. The basic manual on this latter-day version of the laying on of hands by the nurse who developed the approach. The technique is being widely used in orthopedics, presurgery, and primary care, with some startling results in the diminution of pain and improved rate of recovery.

Kuhn, Thomas S. *The Structure of Scientific Revolutions.* 2nd ed. Chicago: University of Chicago Press, 1970. Though not exclusively directed at the issue of science in medicine, this book has become the touchstone for the quest for a "new paradigm" that includes the search for a more holistic medicine.

Kushi, Michio. *Oriental Diagnosis.* London: n.p., 1979. An example of the kind of book that gives holistic medicine a bad name, this slim volume is a minor stew of astrology, snippets of advice on food, and a simplistic manual on facial diagnosis. All the more distressing because the author, a disciple of the "father of macrobiotics," George Ohsawa, is a respected authority on many aspects of Oriental medicine. Strange.

Kuvalayananda, Swami, and Vinekar, S. L. *Yogic Therapy.* New Delhi: Ministry of Health, 1971. Written at the request of the Indian Government in 1961, this book is worth ordering. (Three dollars to Central Health Education Bureau, Ministry of Health, New Delhi, India.) It is a basic and authoritative introduction to Ayruvedic tradition and medical practices.

Lawson-Wood, Denis, and Lawson-Wood, Joyce. *First Aid at Your Fingertips.* Rustington, Sussex, England: Health Sciences Press, 1963. An alphabetical manual of accidents and illnesses treatable by finger acupressure. Telegraphic and direct, with simple line illustrations for determining pressure points.

Leonard, George. *The Silent Pulse.* New York: E. P. Dutton, 1978. In this book Leonard expands the theme of his previous work in the *Ultimate Athlete* to explore rhythm, consciousness, body movement, and the energy phenomena of nature as they relate to well-being and the possibilities of transcendent functioning. Well written and provocative.

LeShan, Lawrence. *How to Meditate.* New York: Bantam Books, 1974. A wonderful, brief, down-to-earth introduction to the principles of meditative practice, with clear instructions on a number of useful beginning exercises that the reader can try without benefit of guru, gobbledegook, or other fancy trappings.

———. *The Mechanic and the Gardener.* New York: Holt, Rinehart and Winston, 1982. Do not be put off by the cryptic title. This is an extremely useful book about such diverse subjects as the relationship of nutrition to medicine, the inextricable connections among body, mind, and spirit, and, for good measure, helpful ways to survive a stay in the hospital. Clear, honest, and authoritative.

Leslie, Charles. *Asian Medical Systems.* Berkeley and Los Angeles: University of California Press, 1976. A collection of fascinating and scholarly papers on aspects of Asian humoral medicine, ranging from general theoretical analysis to specific studies of the social organization of medical practices throughout Asia. A basic and important reference for any serious student.

Li, C. P. *Chinese Herbal Medicine.* Washington, D.C.: Department of Health, Education, and Welfare, 1974. This inexpensive paperback book, one of several Chinese documents translated at the Fogarty International Center for Advanced Study in the Health Sciences, in Washington, is a technical but useful introduction to the complex tradition of using plants for healing. To be read along with Richard Hyatt's book of the same title.

Luce, Gay Gaer. *Bodytime.* New York: Bantam Books, 1973. Still the best popular introduction to the ideas that have given birth to the new field called "chronobiology," the study of the connection between time, physiological and psychological rhythms, and health.

Majno, Guido. *The Healing Hand: Man and Wound in the Ancient World.* Cambridge: Harvard University Press, 1975. The "wound " is merely the inspiration for this lively and exhaustive journey from the beginnings of the physician's art to the modern laboratory. Written with zest and humor, this book is readable as history, science—or as a detective story—about human attempts to conquer pain and disease. Highly recommended.

Mann, Felix. *Acupuncture.* New York: Vintage Books, 1972. One of the best compact summaries of the principles of the basic arm of Chinese medicine, this book contains some provocative statistics on the results of using needles for a wide range of complaints. Serious and instructive.

Maslow, Abraham H. *The Farther Reaches of Human Nature.* New York: Viking Press, 1971. The master's only posthumous book, this collection of his most seminal essays and lectures includes his influential definitions of health, creativity, and values. A vital distillation of the ideas of a psychologist whose theories most influenced the work of the humanistic medicine movement. Can be read and read again with increasing reward.

———. *Motivation and Personality.* 2nd ed. New York: Harper & Row Publishers, 1970. One of the foremost theorists of the humanistic-existential psychologies is noted, among other things, for his courage in defining the "healthy personality." In this, his bedrock textbook, he establishes his famous "hierarchy of needs" and defines health as "growth towards self-actualization." Must be read by anyone who wishes to understand the evolution of the holistic orientation to health and illness.

———. *The Psychology of Science.* New York: Harper & Row Publishers, 1966. One of the best modern interpretations of holism as an attitude toward science. Read along with Polanyi's Personal Knowledge, it provides the best latter-day expansion of Smuts's ideas that wholes are greater than the sum of their parts.

————. *Toward a Psychology of Being.* rev. ed. Princeton, N.J.: Van Nostrand-Reinhold Co., 1968. One of the keystone books in the spread of humanistic psychology and the human potential movement, the antecedent of holistic health. Maslow's definition of the healthy personality lent new authority to seeing health as more than physical well-being, and greatly influenced developments in the use of biofeedback, meditation, mental imagery, and other nonbiomedical approaches to healing. Must be read if you want to understand holistic theory.

Montagu, Ashley. *Touching.* New York: Columbia University Press, 1978. As always in his writing, Montagu is felicitous, convincing, and willing to explore the center of subjects that others only skirt. This book lends new authority to the long-felt conviction that human touch may be the most powerful medicine available to us.

Mumford, Lewis. *The Transformation of Man.* New York: Harper & Row Publishers, 1956. Though this wise philosopher's vast work is not usually associated with issues of medicine or health, this little known but remarkable book is in the mainstream of holistic philosophy and points toward an evolution of both man and nature that includes the perfectibility, not only of institutions and transactions, but of the human mind and body as well. A classic.

Needham, Joseph. *Science and Civilization in China.* 8 vols. Cambridge: At the University Press, 1954–76. Needham is probably the most astute interpreter of Chinese civilization to write for the Western audience. His monumental work has been at the heart of the evolving East-West synthesis that has been emerging in many aspects of the sciences and the humanities.

Ni, Hua-Ching. *Tao: The Subtle Universal Law and the Integral Way of Life.* Los Angeles: Shrine of the Eternal Breath of Tao, 1979. A summary of the Taoist religious, philosophical, and physical worldview, remarkable for the amount of detail covered in brief essays. A useful introduction.

Ohashi, Watari. *Do-It-Yourself Shiatsu.* New York: E. P. Dutton, 1976. A good introduction to the energetic system from Japan that is part massage, part curative acupressure. The author has devised some modern variations on the older technique, but the basis of the system is still energy flow in the meridians.

Ornstein, Robert E. *The Psychology of Consciousness.* San Francisco: W. H. Freeman & Co., 1972. The most readable summary of the research that established the distinctive functions of the two hemispheres of the brain, this book provides a good modern basis for understanding the principles of physiological self-regulation as it has been practiced for centuries in the context of spiritual or Eastern psychological systems.

————, and Naranjo, Claudio. *On the Psychology of Meditation.* New York: Viking Press, 1971. A comprehensive look not only at the mental aspects but also the physiology of meditative practice. Clearly written for a lay audience.

Panos, Maesimund B., and Heimlich, Jane. *Homeopathic Medicine at Home.* Los Angeles: J. P. Tarcher, 1980. The most readable and immediately useful manual of homeopathic medicine, written expressly for the layman. A basic necessity for anyone interested in homeopathy for family self-care.

Pelletier, Kenneth. *Mind as Healer, Mind as Slayer.* New York: Dell Publishing Co., 1977. One of the significant "bridging" books that has helped legitimize the claims of the holistic medicine movement that mind-body interaction can be used by both physician and patient as a central part of therapy and healing. Important, impressive, and readable.

————. *Holistic Medicine: From Stress to Optimum Health.* New York: Seymour Law-rence/Delacorte, 1979. One of the clearest writers and best thinkers about health and illness. Illuminates not only the theories of the holistic medicine movement, but introduces the reader to stress-control techniques, nutritional practices, and exercise strategies that contribute to moving toward dynamic health.

Porkert, Manfred. *The Theoretical Foundations of Chinese Medicine.* Cambridge: MIT Press, 1978. Rigorously scholarly in its approach, which often makes for difficulty in reading, this book is nevertheless rich and comprehensive in its detailed explanation of the "correspondences" that govern Chinese medical theory. Impressive—and essential for the serious student.

Prabhavananda, Swami, and Isherwood, Christopher. *How to Know God: The Yoga Aphorisms of Patanjali.* Hollywood, Calif.: Vedanta Press, 1971. A serious introduction to traditional meditative practices, enhanced by the participation of a gifted English writer, himself a follower of the Vedanta movement.

Remen, Naomi. *The Human Patient.* Garden City, N.Y.: Anchor Press/Doubleday, 1980. A lovely book by a gifted physician and writer who has integrated into medical practice a large variety of techniques aimed at empowering patients to participate more actively in their own self-healing. Draws heavily on principles of Gestalt therapy, mental imagery, transpersonal psychology, and particularly the significance of the *meaning* of illness in the recovery process.

Revolution Health Committee of Hunan Province. *A Barefoot Doctor's Manual: A Guide to Traditional Chinese and Modern Medicine.* DHEW Publication No. (NIH) 75-695. Washington, D.C.: GPO, 1974. Originally published in 1970 in the People's Republic of China, this manual focuses on the improvement of medical and health care facilities in the rural villages of the province as part of the political and social attempt to enlarge the corps of health workers for an expanding population. Technical, but immensely informative, especially the elaborate section on Chinese herbal remedies.

Rogers, Carl E. *On Becoming a Person.* Boston: Houghton Mifflin Co., 1961. This keystone book by one of the most influential American psychologists of the twentieth century has had a deservedly tremendous influence on physicians, particularly because Roger's work with "client-centered" psychotherapy contains so many implications for improving the doctor-patient relationship and the accompanying recovery powers of the sick patient. A classic in the field.

Rolf, Ida. *Rolfing: The Integration of Human Structures.* New York: Harper & Row Publishers, 1978. The Bible of the well-publicized system developed by the author over thirty years. Rolfing, usually a ten-session course of vigorous and deep manipulations of the facial tissues, is credited by many with having profound results on psychophysical health. The debate goes on about its efficacy, but if you would understand the theory in detail, you must read the book.

Rose, Louis. *Faith Healing.* Harmondsworth, Middlesex, England: Penguin Books, 1971. A hardheaded look at the history and some of the modern practices of faith healing by a psychiatrist who, though he could not document the phenomenon to his own satisfaction, remains open—after all his research—to the idea that not all healing or recovery from illness can be explained in "scientific" terms.

Salmon, J. Warren, ed. *Alternative Medicine: Popular and Policy Perspectives.* New York: Tavistock Publications, 1984. A truly unusual symposium that addresses not only the need for the integration of the other medicines into conventional practice, but also describes how such a synthesis will require further reforms of the entire health care system. Several writers also discuss the ticklish, but vital subjects of licensure, reimbursement, and the "corporatization" of health care. An important book.

Samuels, Mike, and Bennett, Hal. *The Well Body Book.* New York: Random House, 1978. The most popular of the heavily illustrated manuals of self-care and health promotion, this book is a good introduction to a broad range of relaxation exercises, fitness programs, and self-regulating treatments, most of them in the "natural" tradition. Attractive and useful.

Sandner, Donald. *Navaho Symbols of Healing.* New York: Harcourt Brace Jovanovich, 1979. A Jungian-trained psychiatrist explores ancient methods of Navajo healing—purification and evocation rites, healing chants, the execution of sand paintings, the rigorous training of the traditional medicine men. Another example of other medicines that work because of a totally different approach to the body-mind relationship. Specialized, but interesting.

Schultz, Johannes Heinrich, and Luthe, Wolfgang. *Autogenic Training.* New York: Grune & Stratton, 1959. The book that introduced a technique of self-regulating exercises of mental imagery and relaxation that in later adapted forms has become part of the general armamentarium of relaxation teachers. Now interesting chiefly for its historic importance.

Sehnert, Keith. *How to Be Your Own Doctor (Sometimes).* New York: Grosset & Dunlap, 1977. A helpful but limited work on self-care by a physician who started the "activated patient" movement, a form of self-care that promotes greater patient education and participation in medical treatment. The treatment, however, is confined to Western medicine.

Selye, Hans. *The Stress of Life.* New York: McGraw-Hill, 1966. A pioneering work that convinced many people of the reality of the effect of stress on health. His discussion on the effects of negative emotions on body chemistry and his persuasive descriptions of the impact of emotional tension on bodily processes were critical.

————. *Stress Without Distress.* Philadelphia: J. B. Lippincott, 1974. An important restatement by the foremost theorist about stress (he coined the word in 1936) in which he argues that an individual's limited adaptational energy is most widely conserved through a philosophy of altruism. Important for its speculations about both physiology and attitudes.

Sharma, Chandra H. *A Manual of Homeopathy and Natural Medicine.* New York: E. P. Dutton, 1976. Another handy and straightforward manual for those interested in homeopathic self-care. Also includes useful, brief background on Hindu medicine.

Shealy, C. Norman. *Ninety Days to Self-Health.* New York: Dial Press, 1977. Shealy is one of the leading physicians in the formal wing of the holistic health movement, and this book summarizes his views on the need for integrating not only the other medicines into health care, but a wide range of promotive techniques with a positive orientation to the possibilities of self-health. Useful, even though the title is more mercantile than accurate.

Shepherd, Dorothy. *Homeopathy for the First Aider.* Rustington, Sussex, England: Health Sciences Press, 1953. A practical, authoritative first aid manual based on the use of homeopathic remedies for accidents, emergencies, and sudden illnesses. Written in a personal, down-to-earth—and convincing—style by a distinguished British homeopath.

Simonton, O. Carl; Mathews-Simonton, Stephanie; and Creighton, James. *Getting Well Again.* Los Angeles: J. P. Tarcher, 1978. A book that stems from the work of the original Simonton team that worked with cancer patients in trying to develop self-regulating techniques to combat the effects of terminal illness. Popular and useful.

Sinnott, Edmund W. *The Biology of the Spirit.* New York: Viking Press, 1955. Sinnott wrote the introduction to the American edition of Smuts's *Holism and Evolution,* but in this work and others he wrote, he made an equally cogent case for broadening the definition of "science" to include matters of the spirit, the soul, and man's undeniable metaphysical yearnings. This book is particularly moving and convincing on that theme.

Siu, R. G. H. *The Tao of Science.* Cambridge: MIT Press, 1964. An early and important attempt to make the case for integrating what the author calls "Western knowledge and Eastern wisdom." A wonderfully clear and convincing, and, unfortunately, neglected work.

Smuts, Jan Christiaan. *Holism and Evolution.* New York: Viking Press, 1961. The work that launched the idea that the striving of organisms for higher and higher levels of organization is the basic evolutionary force in nature—a force he called *"holism."* Indirectly, through the later interpreters of his theory, this book has been one of the most influential of the twentieth century.

Sobel, David S., ed. *Ways of Health.* New York: Harcourt Brace Jovanovich, 1979. This symposium on ancient and modern complementary medical systems includes among its authors some of the most distinguished figures in their fields—René Dubos, Harris Coulter, Herbert Benson, Manfred Porkert, and others—who cover a wide range of topics: Chinese medicine, systems theory, ion therapy, nutrition, Yogic therapy, homeopathy, etc. It is one of the best introductions to holistic medicine for physicians, medical students, and other health care providers.

————, and Hornbacher, Faith. *To Your Health.* New York: Grossman Publishers, 1973. Now out of print, this illustrated manual, taken along with books such as *The Well Body Book,* is a broad and useful introduction to dozens of ways laymen can maintain or improve their health. Contains simple exercises and procedures drawn from dozens of medical and nonmedical systems.

Stanway, Andrew. *Alternative Medicine.* New York: Penguin Books, 1982. A catalogue of thirty-two unconventional therapeutic systems, ranging from anthroposophical medicine to sonic therapy, briefly described and evaluated by a British internist. While limited to those systems that have attracted attention in Great Britain, the book is written clearly and honestly.

Stephenson, James H. *A Doctor's Guide to Helping Yourself with Homeopathic Remedies,* West Nyack, N.Y.: Parker Publishing Co., 1976. A sometimes overenthusiastic manual for self-treatment via homeopathy. Particularly useful for its understandable repertory, but not as well-organized as Panos and Heimlich.

Stuart, Malcolm, ed. *The Encyclopedia of Herbs and Herbals.* New York: Crescent Books, 1977. Originally published in England, this truly encyclopedic book contains sections on the history of herbalism, the biology and chemistry of plants, their medical, kitchen, and cosmetic use, with clear explanations of the cultivation, collection, and preservation of herbs. Beautifully illustrated with color photographs.

Sung Tz'u. *The Washing Away of Wrongs.* Translated by Brian E. McKnight. Ann Arbor: University of Michigan Press, 1981. A new translation of a classic text in forensic medicine originally written in the thirteenth century. Although intended to guide the police pathologist of the time, the chapter on first aid techniques and methods of reviving the dead or unconscious patient are fascinating.

Svensson, Jon-Erik. *Folk Remedies, Receipts, and Advice.* New York: Berkley Publishing Corp., 1977. An affectionate compendium of folklore dealing with health and healing: herbs, medicinal beverages, patent medicines, recipes, and cosmetics. Put together to amuse and entertain, and containing the inevitable nostalgic eighteenth- and nineteenth-century drawings.

Tart, Charles C., ed. *Altered States of Consciousness.* New York: John Wiley & Sons, 1969. An early anthology of articles that explore the relationship between meditation, drugs, and consciousness, and, by extension, health itself.

Taylor, Edmond. *Richer by Asia.* 2nd ed. Boston: Houghton Mifflin Co., 1964. Essentially an appreciation of the richness of Asian history, philosophy, and religion aimed at building an East-West bridge to promote world peace, this book (now available only in libraries) is a brilliantly written exposition of the mind-set that lies behind the Asian medicines. Especially fascinating is the chapter called "The Parable of the Backward Deer," which is a startling critique of what the author calls the "Western Science God."

Thakkur, Chandrashekhar. *Ayurveda: The Indian Art and Science of Medicine.* New York: ASI Publishers, 1974. An attempt to produce an English popularization of the principles of Ayurvedic medicine, with a special emphasis on the Tridosha theory of health and disease. The book suffers from being unevenly written, with sources too casually identified, but it is useful as an introduction to the subject.

Thie, John F. *Touch for Health.* Marina del Rey, Calif.: DeVorss & Co., 1979. The basic manual of the system of the same name, a broad synthesis of chiropractic theory (and the field of applied kinesiology that stemmed from it), massage techniques, and aspects of Oriental acupressure. Particularly useful if the reader has also had at least some workshop training in the system.

Thomas, Lewis. *The Lives of a Cell.* New York: Viking Press, 1974. The first and best-known of three books by one of the premier examples of the cultivated scientist, Thomas is as devoted to the glories of music and poetry as he is to the technical triumphs of scientific medicine, in many of which he has shared personally. Yet, with all the civilized sensibility he possesses, he still persists in seeing his era and his style of medicine as the only one that is truly worthwhile, and he persists in seeing all other formulations of health and medicine as primitive or, at best, irrelevant.

Thomson, William A. R. *Herbs That Heal.* New York: Charles Scribner's Sons, 1977. Though emphasizing the British experience of forsaking medicinal plants for synthetic drugs, this reasoned argument for investigating the therapeutic value of herbs is a careful and readable summary of the issue worldwide.

Tierra, Michael. *The Way of Herbs.* Santa Cruz, Calif.: Unity Press, 1980. A remarkably thorough instructional manual on the use of herbs, both North American and Oriental. Written by a naturopath who is also an acupuncturist, the diagnoses of symptoms relies heavily on Oriental theory, but the book is useful as well for those who seek natural healing agents for common conditions from abscesses to toothaches.

Tillich, Paul. *The Relation of Religion and Health.* Richmond, Calif.: North Atlantic Books, 1982. A book-length version of a classical essay by the late theologian whose ideas have profoundly influenced the existential branch of modern psychology. Here he establishes the convincing connection between "healing" and "salvation," an argument that demands that the biological and spiritual sides of man be united if he is to be truly healthy. See also his great work *The Courage to Be.*

Vickery, Donald M., and Fries, James F. *Take Care of Yourself: A Consumer's Guide to Medical Care.* Reading, Mass.: Addison-Wesley Publishing Co., 1979. An excellent manual for laymen containing simplified, comprehensible charts for the diagnosis and treatment of common medical problems from arthritis to toothaches.

Veith, Ilza, trans. *Huang Ti Nei Ching Su Wen (The Yellow Emperor's Classic of Internal Medicine).* Chaps. 1–34. Berkeley and Los Angeles: University of California Press, 1972. An easily readable translation of a sizable segment of one of the most important theoretical texts in Chinese medical literature. The introductory material by the translator is invaluable in orienting the Western reader to the breadth of thought that underlies Chinese medical practice.

Vogel, Virgil J. *American Indian Medicine.* Norman: University of Oklahoma Press, 1970. A comprehensive and detailed survey of a vast field, this book is becoming a classic in medical anthropology. Now in its fourth printing, it bids fair to be the cornerstone book on the subject. Scholarly, greatly detailed, but fascinating and readable for the serious student.

Wallis, Roy, and Morley, Peter, eds. *Culture and Curing.* London: Peter Owen, 1978. A group of essays on the connection between cultural beliefs and attitudes toward health and illness. Spiritualist healing, magic ritual, tribal custom, and folklore are all explored by anthropologists and sociologists. Primarily of interest to scholars.

————, eds. *Marginal Medicine.* New York: Free Press, 1976. A series of essays about the relationship between unorthodox medicine and society, providing a sound anthropological and sociological explanation for the persistence of "alternative medicine" in the midst of a "scientific" society.

Weil, Andrew. *The Marriage of the Sun and Moon.* Boston: Houghton Mifflin Co., 1980. A delightfully written account of the author's journeys in North and South America in a quest to understand the connections between plants and consciousness. His experiences with everything from cocaine to mushrooms have immense implications for our ideas about health and the mind-body connection. Fascinating, as is his other book, *The Natural Mind.*

————. *Health and Healing: Understanding Conventional and Alternative Medicine.* Boston: Houghton Mifflin Co., 1984. A personal, well-written, and bold interpretation of the meaning of human health and illness by one of the most astute physicians writing today. The book is also an eloquent and persuasive argument for paying serious attention to such medical "unorthodoxies" as homeopathy, naturopathy, Chinese medicine, and even shamanism.

Weiner, Michael, and Goss, Kathleen. *The Complete Book of Homeopathy.* New York: Bantam Books, 1982. Ranks with Panos and Heimlich's *Homeopathic Medicine at Home* as one of the books that makes the principles and practice of homeopathy most accessible to the layman. Seriously but clearly written.

Welch, Holmes. *Taoism.* Boston: Beacon Press, 1965. Read along with the books by John Blofeld, this small volume gives the Western lay reader the best general introduction to the Chinese philosophical system that most influenced the development of Oriental medicine. Scholarly, civilized, near poetic in places, this little book is pure pleasure.

Welwood, John, ed. *The Meeting of the Ways: Explorations in East/West Psychology.* New York: Schocken Books, 1979. A particularly useful anthology on the movement toward fusion of the Eastern traditions of Taoism, Hinduism, Buddhism, and Sufism and the Western commitment to science and technology. Especially relevant are the contributions that look at the potential usefulness of meditation and other consciousness-altering techniques to therapy.

Werner, David. *Where There Is No Doctor.* Palo Alto, Calif.: Hesperian Foundation, 1977. A remarkable handbook designed expressly for village health workers in Latin America who have had no formal medical training. Clear, complete instructions for dealing with everything from emergencies and first aid to childbirth. Virtually encyclopedic, and easy to use. Available most readily by mail order: P.O. Box 1692, Palo Alto, Calif. 94302.

Whitmont, Edward C. *Psyche and Substance.* Richmond, Calif.: North Atlantic Books, 1980. A group of essays written over twenty-five years by a distinguished Jungian psychoanalyst who is also a practicing homeopath. His speculations on the mind-body relationship, relying heavily on Jungian symbolism, are provocative and inspiring. A superb example of truly holistic thinking.

Williams, Roger J. *Biochemical Individuality.* New York: John Wiley & Sons, 1956. The technical introduction to the theories of the man who has become the nutrition "guru" of the holistic health movement. Williams's belief in physiological individuality forms the perfect basis for emphasis on self-responsibility and self-care. (The more popularly written book on the subject is the author's *Nutrition Against Disease.)*

Wilson, Judy. *Mother Nature's Homestead First Aid.* Willits, Calif.: Oliver Press, 1975. One of a series of manuals published at the height of the back-to-the-country movement, this brief manual is a useful guide for those who live or work far from formal medical services. It features improvisational techniques for accidents that can occur anywhere.

Yin Wing Choi. *The Topography of Fourteen Meridians.* South Pasadena, Calif.: n.p., 1973. A technical but clear introduction to the essence of the basic meridians and their relationship to the internal organs. One hundred fifty of the 360 classically designated acupuncture points are described and handsomely illustrated in simple color charts.

Zimmer, Henry R. *Hindu Medicine.* Baltimore: Johns Hopkins University Press, 1948. The most accessible Western interpretation of the underpinnings of Ayurvedic and Yogic therapeutics, by a distinguished scholar who understood the cultural and religious roots of Hinduism as well as medical techniques. Readable and scholarly in equal measure.

INDEX